New Technologies in Clinical Laboratory Science

New Technologies in Clinical Laboratory Science

Edited by
N. K. Shinton
with the assistance of E. A. Gloag

Proceedings of the fifth ECCLS Seminar
held at Siena, Italy, 23–25 May 1984

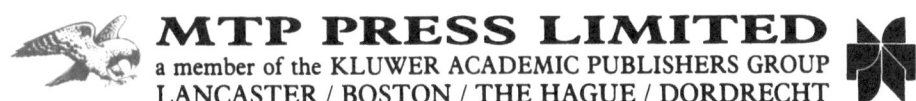

MTP PRESS LIMITED
a member of the KLUWER ACADEMIC PUBLISHERS GROUP
LANCASTER / BOSTON / THE HAGUE / DORDRECHT

Published in the UK and Europe by
MTP Press Limited
Falcon House
Lancaster, England

British Library Cataloguing in Publication Data

New technologies in clinical laboratory science.
  1. Diagnosis, Laboratory
  I. Shinton, N. K. II. Gloag, E. A.
  616.07'5   RB37

Published in the USA by
MTP Press
A division of Kluwer Boston Inc
190 Old Derby Street
Hingham, MA 02043, USA

Library of Congress Cataloging in Publication Data

Main entry under title:

New technologies in clinical laboratory science.

   Papers presented at a meeting held in May 1984 in
Siena, Italy, sponsored by the European Committee for
Clinical Laboratory Standards.
   Includes bibliographies and index.
   1. Diagnosis, Laboratory—Congresses. 2. Nuclear
magnetic resonance—Congresses. 3. Deoxyribonucleic
acid—Analysis—Congresses. 4. Antibodies, Monoclonal—
Congresses. 5. Biosensors—Congresses. I. Shinton, N. K.
(Keith) II. Gloag, E. A. (Ann) III. European Committee
for Clinical Laboratory Standards. [DNLM: 1. Antibodies,
Monoclonal—congresses. 2. Biochemistry—methods—
congresses. 3. DNA, Recombinant—congresses. 4. Nuclear
Magnetic Resonance—congresses. QU 25 N532 1984]
RB37.A2N49 1985   616.07'5   85-24236

ISBN-13: 978-94-010-8684-4   e-ISBN-13: 978-94-009-4928-7
DOI: 10.1007/978-94-009-4928-7

Typeset by Blackpool Typesetting Services Limited

Contents

v

Preface

As with the previous four ECCLS Seminars, the contributions to the fifth Seminar in Siena have been collected together for the benefit both of those who were fortunate to be present and those unable to come. This Seminar differed from the others in having a more purely scientific content; however the contributors also considered the possible need for standardization in the future. The speakers were chosen for their acknowledged expertise in the specific topics. The papers are now presented in the order in which they were given with editorial change only to give consistency of style of presentation. It follows that each paper can stand alone at the expense of a minimum of repetition. Because the topics are in rapidly developing fields of high technology, speed of publication was essential; for help with this, ECCLS thanks the contributors.

List of Contributors

W. H. W. ALBERT
Boehringer Mannheim GMBH
Biochemical Research Centre
D-8132 Tutzing
Federal Republic of Germany

D. M. BAND
Sherrington School of Physiology
St Thomas Hospital Medical School
Lambeth Palace Road
London SE1 7EH
United Kingdom

D. AMMAN
Department of Organic Chemistry
Swiss Federal Institute of
  Technology (ETH)
Universitätstr. 16
CH-8092 Zurich
Switzerland

M. L. BIANCHI BANDINELLI
Institute of Microbiology
University of Siena
Via Laterina 8
53100 Siena
Italy

P. ANKER
Department of Organic Chemistry
Swiss Federal Institute of
  Technology (ETH)
Universitätstr. 16
CH-8092 Zurich
Switzerland

P. O. BRUNNER
Medical Instruments
Spectrospin AG
Industriestrasse 26
CH-8117 Fällanden
Switzerland

D. ARMELLINI
Sclavo Research Centre
53100 Siena
Italy

M. BUGNOLI
Sclavo Research Centre
53100 Siena
Italy

A. BUSSARD
Department of Immunology
Medical School
Avenue de Vallombrose
06034 Nice
France

A. K. COVINGTON
Electrochemistry Research
   Laboratories
Department of Physical Chemistry
University of Newcastle upon Tyne
Newcastle upon Tyne NE1 7RU
United Kingdom

M. L. DI CAIRANO
Institute of Microbiology
University of Siena
Via Laterina 8
53100 Siena
Italy

G. DOUGAN
Molecular Biology/Bacterial
   Genetics
Wellcome Research Laboratories
Langley Court
Beckenham, Kent
United Kingdom

A. FERRIDGE
Physical Chemistry Department
Wellcome Research Laboratories
Langley Court
Beckenham, Kent
United Kingdom

D. G. GADIAN
Physics in Relation to Surgery
The Royal College of Surgeons of
   England
35–43 Lincoln's Inn Fields
London WC2A 3PN
United Kingdom

E. GAGGELLI
Department of Chemistry
University of Siena
Via Pian dei Mantellini 44
53100 Siena
Italy

F. GÜTTLER
John F. Kennedy Instituttet
Gl. Landevej 7
DK-2600 Glostrup
Denmark

A. HENREN
Department of Biotechnology
Ciba-Geigy AG
CH-4002 Basel
Switzerland

P. HIGHFIELD
Diagnostics R & D
Wellcome Research Laboratories
Langley Court
Beckenham, Kent BR3 3BS
United Kingdom

P. LEONCINI
Sclavo Research Centre
53100 Siena
Italy

A. MASSONE
Sclavo Research Centre
53100 Siena
Italy

A. TIEZZI
Sclavo Research Centre
53100 Siena
Italy

V. PALLINI
Sclavo Research Centre
53100 Siena
Italy

G. VALENSIN
Department of Chemistry
University of Siena
Via Pian dei Mantellini 44
53100 Siena
Italy

H. RUDOLPH
Department of Biotechnology
Ciba-Geigy AG
CH-4002 Basel
Switzerland

P. RUGGIERO
Sclavo Research Centre
53100 Siena
Italy

P. E. VALENSIN
Institute of Microbiology
University of Siena
Via Laterina 8
53100 Siena
Italy

G. SCAPIGLIATI
Sclavo Research Centre
53100 Siena
Italy

W. SIMON
Department of Organic Chemistry
Swiss Federal Institute of
   Technology (ETH)
Universitätstr. 16
CH-8092 Zürich
Switzerland

M. WINTHER
Department of Microbial
   Development
Wellcome Biotechnology Ltd
Langley Court
Beckenham, Kent BR3 3BS
United Kingdom

Part 1
NUCLEAR MAGNETIC RESONANCE

1
Theoretical and technical aspects of nuclear magnetic resonance

A. FERRIGE

For practical purposes the history of nuclear magnetic resonance (NMR) goes back only to late 1945 when Block and Purcell independently observed NMR signals for the first time. It was not until the mid-1960s that commercial instruments became readily available, and prior to this many workers built their own equipment.

In simple terms all magnetically active nuclei will absorb radiowaves when immersed in a magnetic field. Nuclei behave like micromagnets and some orient in the direction of the field and precess at a specific frequency. Following spontaneous excitation by a burst or pulse of radiowaves of the correct frequency, the detected amplitude versus time signal is that emitted as the nuclei lose energy by 'relaxing' back to their original state. The complex mixture of decaying frequencies is Fourier transformed to produce an amplitude versus frequency trace which is much more readily interpreted by the scientist. However, for a fixed magnetic field the frequency of signals varies by very small amounts depending on the chemical environment of the different nuclei present, and at a magnetic field of 2.35 Tesla hydrogen nuclei (protons) resonate at 100 MHz with a frequency variation rarely exceeding 15 ppm. At the same field carbon-13 nuclei resonate at approximately 25 MHz with a spread of approximately 200 ppm.

Almost all elements have at least one magnetically active isotope but for many the sensitivity is very low. However, operation at higher magnetic fields, and correspondingly higher frequencies, yields large gains in the sensitivity, selectivity and peak discrimination. The development of a whole new magnet technology based on liquid

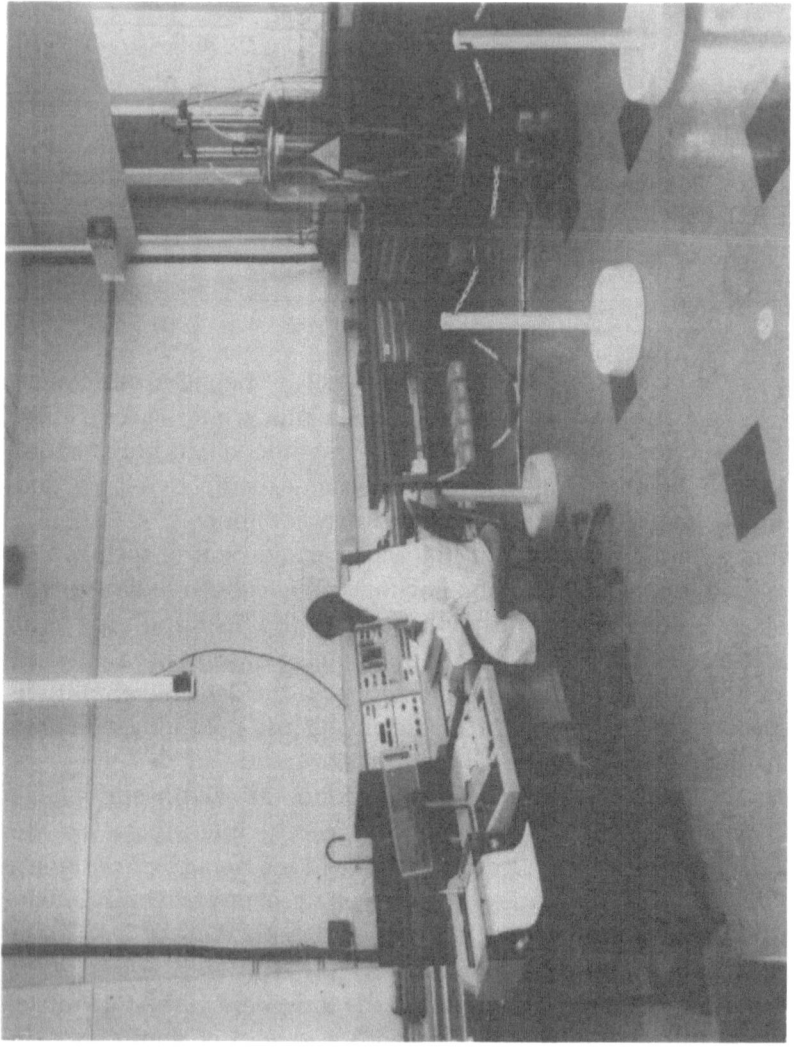

Figure 1.1   A typical high resolution NMR spectrometer

helium superconducting solenoids which now generate fields of the order of 12 Tesla has enabled many of the less sensitive nuclei to be investigated routinely and the list of usable elements has been extended from ^1H, ^{19}F and ^{31}P to include ^{23}Na, ^{13}C and ^{15}N.

Molecules in solution produce sharp, well-defined resonances as opposed to solids where signals are very broad. The technique has therefore been most widely used traditionally by organic chemists to probe chemical structure. Modern instruments, however, allow the operator almost infinite flexibility to manipulate nuclei prior to signal detection so that only relevant data are collected. Iain Campbell of the Oxford Enzyme Group has been a pioneer of such methods[1] and has applied them using proton, carbon and phosphorus to enzyme kinetics and studies on intact cells[2]. The proton spectra of large molecules such as haemoglobin and membranes are broad and ill-defined, but by adopting special radio frequency pulse sequences broad-signal components are eliminated, allowing weak, sharp resonances from metabolites to be observed and quantified.

A natural extension of this work to the examination of metabolic processes and reaction kinetics in perfused organs followed, and many laboratories now regularly perfuse hearts, kidneys etc. in NMR spectrometers in order to observe the effect of potential therapeutic molecules on metabolism. Such procedures have the benefit of using the same organ for both the experiment and the control, thus inter-animal variations are less critical and the need for experimental animals is reduced.

Early work at Oxford demonstrated the value of NMR as a quality control tool for kidney transplants by determining the energy status of donor kidneys. The work on cells and organs also revealed that intracellular pH may be accurately determined from phosphorus spectra by measuring the position of the inorganic phosphate signal and this later proved to be, along with other spectral features, an invaluable probe for investigating metabolic disorders *in vivo*.

The inventiveness of academic and industrial scientists has forced magnet technology to develop, and large-bore magnets were produced capable of accepting mice or small rats. New surface coil detection systems were developed to receive signals from a localized area and it became possible to study metabolism *in vivo* in organs such as the brain and muscles. The study of human arms during exercise[3] and rest was made possible by even larger magnets and Radda pioneered the investigation of high-energy phosphate metabolism as a function of metabolic and other disorders. Such studies on patients have included NADH-coenzyme Q reductase deficiency[4], myophosphorylase deficiency (McArdle's syndrome)[5], phosphofructokinase deficiency[6] and Duchenne dystrophy[7].

^{1}H and ^{31}P NMR are now used to investigate cerebral metabolism in newborn infants. Wilkie *et al.* have used this technique to detect birth asphyxia and monitor the effect of treatment[8]. They have also observed left and right hemispheres separately. In one case the loss of brain tissue and impaired energy status in the left hemisphere of an infant was detected at a very early stage. It was later confirmed by ultrasound which showed porencephalic cysts.

In parallel with all the above techniques Mansfield, Andrew and others were pursuing NMR imaging. Here use is made of the different rates at which nuclei, normally the proton, lose energy to their surroundings following the burst of exciting radiowaves. This is primarily governed by molecular size and motion and by employing special pulse sequences and sophisticated mathematical processing these differences are easily resolved spatially. Hence it is possible to examine sections of the human anatomy and three-dimensional images can be constructed from two-dimensional slices. New whole-body magnets now allow any part of the patient to be studied non-invasively.

NMR imaging complements X-ray tomography in that NMR most successfully observes soft tissues whilst X-ray techniques are receptive to hard tissue and bone. By applying different algorithms during data processing images can be 'tuned' to specific relaxation rates or the contrast enhanced to obtain further information. Imaging techniques have been used to detect subdural haematoma[9], brain glyomas and extent of oedema[9], breast cancer and lung cancer.

The 'state of the art' imaging instruments are now capable of observing blood flows and rates from the heart and detecting heart defects such as uraemic pericarditis which is normally only discovered at autopsy[9]. They are also able to produce spectra of any part of the human anatomy and hence non-invasive metabolic and kinetic studies are now a reality[10].

The continued rapid growth of NMR and its wide appeal make it impossible to predict the future. However, there can be little doubt that the next few years will see the technique become a routine medical diagnostic tool.

ACKNOWLEDGEMENTS

The assistance of the following scientists and manufacturers in providing material for this paper is gratefully acknowledged. W. Ammann, Varian Associates; I. Campbell, Oxford Enzyme Group; J. A. Deegan, Diasonics; D. Gadian, Oxford Enzyme Group; R. Gordon, Oxford Research Systems; V. I. P. Jones, Bruker Spectrospin; G. Radda, Radda Group, Oxford; D. Shaw, General Electric; P. Styles, Radda Group, Oxford; D. Wilkie, University College, London.

REFERENCES

1. Campbell, I. D. (1977). *FEBS Lett.*, **82**, 12–16
2. Campbell, I. D. (private communication)
3. Radda, G. K. *et al.* (1983). *Mol. Biol. Med.*, **1**, 77–94
4. Radda, G. K. *et al.* (1982). *Nature*, **295**, 608–9
5. Radda, G. K. *et al.* (1981). *Nature*, **304**, 1338–42
6. Wilkie, D. R. *et al.* (1982). *Lancet*, 725–31
7. Radda G. K. *et al.* (1982). *Br. Med. J.*, **284**, 1072–4
8. Wilkie, D. R. *et al.* (1983). *Lancet*, 1059–62
9. Deegan, J. A. Diasonics (private communication)
10. Bottomlay, B. A. (1983). *Lancet*, 273–4

2
Nuclear magnetic resonance studies of metabolism *in vivo*

D. G. GADIAN

This article briefly reviews the type of information that nuclear magnetic resonance (NMR) can provide about metabolism in living systems. The work of several laboratories will be discussed, and further details of these studies can be found in the general references that are listed at the end of the article.

The nuclei that have been most widely used for metabolic studies are ^{13}C and ^{31}P, but it seems likely that ^{1}H and perhaps ^{19}F NMR will also become increasingly important for studies of this type. If we firstly consider the ^{31}P NMR spectra of intact tissues, the signals that are most commonly observed are from the three phosphate groups of ATP, inorganic phosphate, and in the case of muscle and brain, phosphocreatine. In addition, signals are frequently detected from sugar phosphates, phosphodiesters, and NAD. The simplicity of the spectra reflects the fact that narrow signals are observed only from mobile phosphorus-containing compounds that are present at concentrations above about 0.2 mmol/l; highly immobilized compounds such as membrane phospholipids produce very broad signals, which often show up in the spectrum as a sloping baseline, while compounds that are present at concentrations below 0.2 mmol/l produce weak signals that may be lost in the noise. If ADP were present in mobile form at sufficiently high concentration, it would generate two signals overlapping with the signals from the γ and α phosphates of ATP. It is of considerable interest that ADP generally makes no detectable contribution to the spectra of well-oxygenated tissues, suggesting that the concentration of free ADP is very much lower than the total amounts that are estimated by the technique of

9

freeze-clamping. It is similarly of interest that the concentration of inorganic phosphate as measured by NMR is generally lower than values obtained using other methods. A possible explanation for these discrepancies is that the more traditional invasive methods involve an unavoidable breakdown of high-energy phosphates. In addition, it could be that significant quantities of these metabolites are bound in such a way (e.g. to muscle myofilaments) that the bound fraction generates no detectable signal.

A particularly useful feature of the spectra is that the frequency of the inorganic phosphate signal is sensitive to pH variations in the physiological range. This signal therefore provides a monitor of intracellular pH. The sensitivity to pH arises because the state of ionization of inorganic phosphate changes in the physiological range (the compound has a pK_a of about 6.75). In addition, the frequencies of the ATP signals are sensitive to the binding of divalent metal ions. On the basis of titrations performed *in vitro*, it can be concluded that the ATP within tissues is predominantly complexed to divalent metal ions, presumably Mg^{2+} ions. This conclusion is of interest because the state of ATP *in vivo* has a considerable influence on its biological activity, and also because it enables information to be obtained about the concentration of free Mg^{2+} *in vivo*.

The concentrations of the various metabolites are, under certain conditions, proportional to the areas of their respective signals, and therefore metabolic processes can be followed simply by monitoring how the signal areas vary with time. However, it should be noted that careful controls are necessary in order to quantify the concentrations of metabolites, particularly in studies where there may be some uncertainty as to precisely where within the sample the signal is coming from. The time resolution of the method depends on a large number of factors, but for many studies it is a few minutes. Sometimes spectra can be obtained in as little as 15 seconds, and for some experiments the time resolution can be greatly enhanced by synchronizing the collection of data with physiological activity.

NMR can readily be used in this way to follow the changes in metabolite levels and pH that are associated with muscular contraction, ischaemia, etc., and numerous studies have been described (see references at end of article). However, under most circumstances the metabolic state of a tissue will remain constant with time. What information can NMR provide about this steady state? In addition to providing a non-invasive method of monitoring metabolite levels and intracellular pH, NMR also enables us to measure the rates of certain reactions taking place under steady-state conditions. In one type of experiment a magnetic label in the form of a suitable isotope can be added to the sample, and the metabolic fate of this label can be followed simply by monitoring the spectra as a function of time. This forms the basis of many ^{13}C NMR studies, as described below. In the second type of experiment, termed saturation transfer NMR, no exogenous label is introduced. Instead, a type of 'magnetic labelling' is achieved by using the NMR spectrometer to alter the magnetic properties of a given compound. Saturation transfer measurements have provided some very interesting results about the activity of creatine kinase *in vivo*.

Moving on to nuclei other than ^{31}P, the abundant isotope of carbon, ^{12}C, has no magnetic properties and does not produce NMR signals. Therefore ^{13}C, which is only 1% abundant, is used. In order to obtain detectable signals, the compounds under observation must be highly concentrated (e.g. glycogen in liver, or fats). Otherwise it is necessary to enrich the sample with ^{13}C-labelled material, and in this way it is possible to perform ^{13}C NMR studies that are analogous in many respects to radioactive tracer studies using ^{14}C. ^{13}C NMR has an advantage over ^{31}P NMR that in principle a much larger range of compounds is amenable to study. However, the scope of the technique is at present limited by the large amounts of ^{13}C-label that must be used, and by the price of such amounts of suitably labelled compounds.

^{1}H NMR is much more sensitive than ^{31}P or ^{13}C NMR, and therefore in favourable circumstances it can detect metabolites that are present at concentrations below 0.2 mmol/l. In addition, because of the ubiquity of the hydrogen atom, very many compounds are in principle accessible to study. However, this ubiquity also leads to problems: firstly because the spectra may contain so many overlapping signals that they defy interpretation, but also because water (and sometimes fats) produces an enormous signal that can mask the signals of interest. These problems have been overcome for studies of cellular suspensions, and at least to some extent have now been overcome for intact tissues and whole animals. ^{1}H NMR studies of metabolism could prove to be most fruitful.

Although the large ^{1}H signal from water is a nuisance in studies of metabolism, it can of course be used to great advantage in NMR imaging, as demonstrated in one or two of the accompanying articles.

Many studies have been performed on isolated tissues. Extension to whole animals and humans relied on the development of (a) wide-bore magnets with the homogeneity and field strength required for metabolic studies, and (b) methods of focusing or localizing on a particular region of interest within the animal or human. At the time of writing, suitable magnets that are large enough to accommodate human limbs or neonates have been available for about 3 years, whereas whole-body systems have only just become available. For this reason many of the human studies so far described have been of the forearm. In particular, ^{31}P NMR spectra have been observed from forearm muscle at rest, during exercise and during recovery, both in control subjects and in patients with muscle disorders. There is not scope in this article to discuss the results that have been obtained, but these studies have been discussed by Radda *et al.* (see references).

With regard to methods of localization, the spatial selectivity provided by surface coils has greatly extended the scope of metabolic studies, and focusing on internal organs has been achieved with magnetic field profiling, but further improvements need to be made; this is an important area of current research. However, regardless of the method that is employed, it must be appreciated that the spatial resolution for metabolic studies will be very much poorer than for proton imaging. This is primarily because the concentrations of the metabolites under investigation are typically a few millimolar, whereas the water protons that provide the basis for proton imaging are present at concentrations of up to 100 mol/l.

^{31}P NMR is being used to study cerebral metabolism in newborn infants, and following the recent installation of whole body systems, spectra of the adult head have now been obtained. At this stage, however, it is difficult to predict the eventual scope of such studies. They should certainly enhance our understanding of the metabolism of healthy and diseased tissue, and of the response to therapy. However, it remains to be seen whether these metabolic studies will be used purely at a research level, or whether they will find more routine application in clinical medicine.

GENERAL REFERENCES

There is not space in this brief article to give the many original references relating to the studies that I have discussed. However, the book and review articles given below between them provide the relevant references and discuss many of the topics in detail.

Alger, J. R. and Shulman, R. G. (1984). Metabolic applications of high-resolution ^{13}C nuclear magnetic resonance spectroscopy. *Br. Med. Bull.*, **40**, 160–4

Gadian, D. G. (1982). *Nuclear Magnetic Resonance and its Applications to Living Systems*. (Oxford: Oxford University Press)

Gadian, D. G. (1983). Whole organ metabolism studied by NMR. *Ann. Rev. Biophys. Bioeng.*, **12**, 69–89

Radda, G. K., Bore, P. J. and Rajagopalan, B. (1984). Clinical aspects of ^{31}P NMR spectroscopy. *Br. Med. Bull.*, **40**, 155–9

In addition, the following original articles illustrate some of the topics that may be of particular interest.

Behar, K. L., den Hollander, J. A., Stromski, M. E., Ogino, T., Shulman, R. G., Petroff, O. A. C. and Prichard, J. W. (1983). High-resolution ^{1}H nuclear magnetic resonance study of cerebral hypoxia *in vivo*. *Proc. Natl. Acad. Sci. USA*, **80**, 4945–8

Cady, E. B., Dawson, M. Joan, Hope, P. L., Tofts, P. S., Costello, A. M. de L., Delphy, D. T., Reynolds, E. O. R. and Wilkie, D. R. (1983). Non-invasive investigation of cerebral metabolism in newborn infants by phosphorus nuclear magnetic resonance spectroscopy. *Lancet*, **1**, 1059–62

Shoubridge, E. A., Briggs, R. W. and Radda, G. K. (1982). ^{31}P NMR saturation transfer measurements of the steady state rates of creatine kinase and ATP synthetase in the rat brain. *FEBS Lett.*, **140**, 288–92

Taylor, D. J., Bore, P. J., Styles, P., Gadian, D. G. and Radda, G. K. (1983). Bioenergetics of intact human muscle. A ^{31}P nuclear magnet resonance study. *Mol. Biol. Med.*, **1**, 77–94

3
Virus-infected cells studied by nuclear magnetic resonance

P. E. VALENSIN, G. VALENSIN,
M. L. BIANCHI BANDINELLI, M. L. DI CAIRANO
and E. GAGGELLI

The physiological and pathological properties of living cells and tissues, including malignancy, have been often investigated by means of nuclear magnetic resonance (NMR) behaviour of water in biological systems[1-7]. In fact, the proton relaxation times, T_1 and T_2, are closely related to the dynamic parameter τ_c which characterizes the molecular reorientational motions.

$$\frac{1}{T_1} = \frac{6}{10} \frac{\gamma^4 \hbar^2}{r^6} \left(\frac{\tau}{1 + \omega_0^2 \tau^2} + \frac{4\tau}{1 + 4\omega_0^2 \tau^2} \right)$$

$$\frac{1}{T_2} = \frac{3}{10} \frac{\gamma^4 \hbar^2}{r^6} \left(3 + \frac{5\tau}{1 + \omega_0^2 \tau^2} + \frac{2\tau}{1 + 4\omega_0^2 \tau^2} \right)$$

The first part of the equations gives the size of the magnetic interaction responsible for relaxation (ω_0 is the resonance frequency, $\hbar$ is Planck's universal constant).

Although several investigations and theoretical interpretations have been attempted[3, 4, 8-12], a unique model of the physical state of water in biological systems has not been provided. However the absence of such an interpretation does not impede the use of NMR parameters as markers of the physiological or pathological state.

The most striking observation from the NMR of water in biological systems is that malignant tissues are characterized by longer T_1 times when compared to healthy tissues of the same organ[6, 13, 14].

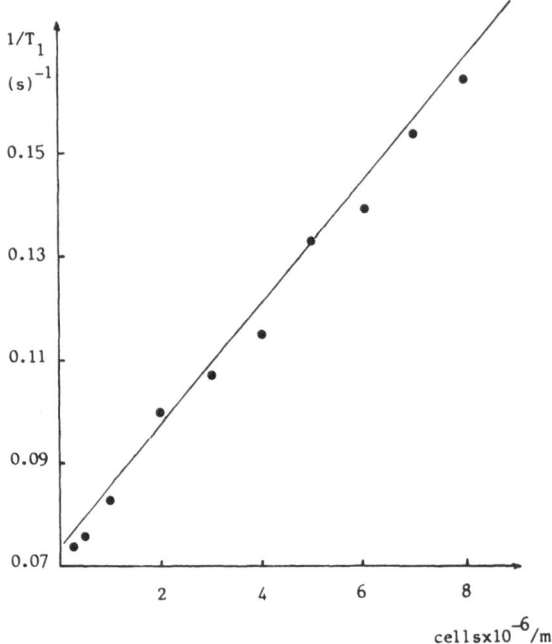

Figure 3.1   Spin–lattice relaxation rates of cell water protons against the cell concentration[15]

HEp-2 cell suspensions in deuterated phosphate buffered saline display a simple exponential decay of the longitudinal magnetization which fits a single T_1 value. When measuring the water proton relaxation rate in cell cultures, shown in Fig. 3.1, a linear relationship is apparent between the $1/T_1$ value and the cell concentration.

However, due to the poor reliability of the cell counting, and also because of the possible physiological modifications of the cells, different T_1 values can be found for apparently equal concentrations, so that it is not possible to know the T_1 value from the cell concentration or vice-versa. According to these findings results from different cell preparations cannot be directly compared; each experiment must thus have its own reference control, that is a strictly homogeneous cell sample.

The observation that the time evolution of cell cultures *in vitro* could be suitably checked by NMR spectroscopy was the starting point for our research project on NMR detection of virus-infected cells. The first efforts have been dedicated to setting up standard procedures for NMR experiments with virus-infected cells. It was a relatively easy task since the infectious process brings about a fast modification of the cell water T_1. In fact a detectable NMR signal (that is to say an appreciable change in T_1) can be obtained within 1 h of virus–cell contact. Moreover the following four statements could be made from experimental evidence during our investigations of the virus-induced T_1 changes in cell cultures: the T_1 measured 1 h after adsorption with viral preparations at 37 °C (a) *changes* (i) in relation to the multiplicity of infection, (ii) in relation to virion structure; (b) *does not change* (i) when lacking specific receptors for virus adsorption, (ii) when viruses are previously neutralized by specific antibodies.

(a-i)   The NMR signal is very specific since the T_1 change is strictly related to the multiplicity of infection[16, 17]. It must be said, at this point, that NMR experiments with viruses at high cytocidal activity, such as poliovirus and vaccinia virus, do not yield any improvement in sensitivity as compared with other virological techniques. In fact, as shown in Fig. 3.2, in poliovirus-infected HEp-2 cells, the lowest multiplicity of infection causing productive infection (10^{-5} PFU/cell) is just that corresponding to the limit of observable T_1 changes; with the vaccinia virus the limit corresponds to 10^{-4} PFU/cell in both cases. However the time saving (1 h against 6 days) is still worth considering.

(a-ii)   The second point is that the structure of virions (naked or enveloped) determines the mode of penetration into the host cell, and this results in different water T_1 changes. It is easily recognized in Table 3.1 that after 1 h of contact at 37 °C the same multiplicities of infection of three naked viruses (polio, coxsackie, adenovirus) shorten the water T_1, while those of four enveloped viruses (Herpes simplex, measles, respiratory syncytial virus, vaccinia virus) lengthen the cell water T_1. In the same way it can be shown that another enveloped virus, the rabies virus, induces lengthening of the tissue water T_1 in vivo.

(b-i)   The third point is that the change in T_1 reflects the viral interaction with specific cell receptors since no effect could be detected when adsorbing rabbit RK-13 cells with poliovirus.

(b-ii)   The fourth point seems the most important. The virus-induced NMR signal can be neutralized by virus-specific antibody; in other

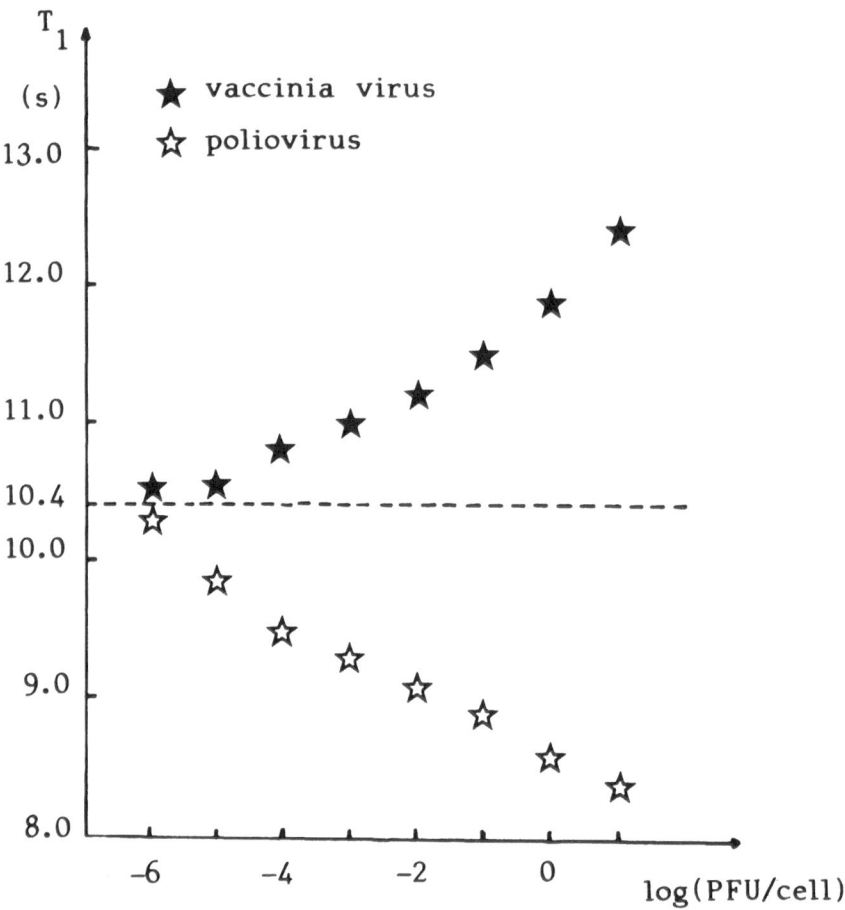

Figure 3.2   Water proton T_1 in HEp-2 cells 1 h after infection vs PFU/cell ratios of poliovirus type 1 and vaccinia virus. Each sample contained 1×10^6 cells. The dashed line gives the cell water T_1 in the cell control[17]

words keeping viruses and antibodies in contact, at proper dilutions and times, prevents the change in water T_1 which otherwise is an early indication of viral infection. These first experiments demonstrate that NMR detection of virus infection is reproducible, specific, fast and easy to perform.

Table 3.1 Cell water T_1 in HEp-2 cell cultures (10^6 cells) after 1 h adsorption with different viruses (0.1 PFU/cell)[17]

Sample	T_1 (s)
Cell control	9.4
Poliovirus type 1	7.1
Coxsackievirus B-3	7.3
Adenovirus	8.0
Measles virus	10.6
Respiratory syncytial virus	12.3
Herpes simplex subtype 1	11.4
Vaccinia virus	10.9

More recent research has been directed towards two different aims: one is the eventual application of NMR spectroscopy to virological diagnosis, the other is the possibility of shedding further light on the relationship between NMR behaviour of cell water and evolution of viral infection. The results obtained up to now, though not conclusive, are very promising and show that further efforts in both directions are really deserved.

Let us consider first the serological diagnosis which is easily worked out in virological laboratories, although the results are not always very useful for clinicians. Since it is easy to have viral strains propagated in laboratory which, when infecting host cells, yield specific and reproducible NMR signals neutralized by homologue antibodies, a serological NMR diagnosis can be suitably pursued. This has been done with many viruses; two examples dealing with a naked virus (poliovirus type 1) and an enveloped one (Herpes simplex virus type 1) are shown in Table 3.2. In both cases it may be recognized that neutralization of viral infectivity and neutralization of virus-induced NMR signals are very closely related.

As far as direct diagnosis is concerned, its clinical importance, and the fact that it is generally quite a difficult process, deserve a more comprehensive discussion. It is important here to underline that, when studying viruses with poor cytocidal activity, the NMR method is more sensitive than common virological techniques. In the case of respiratory syncytial virus, shown in Table 3.3, the NMR measurements

Table 3.2   Cell water T_1 in HEp-2 cell cultures (10^6 cells) after 1 h adsorption with P-1 and HSV-1 (0.1 PFU/cell) in the presence of the corresponding specific antiserum previously adsorbed on HEp-2 cells[17]

Sample	T_1 (s)	CPE[a]
HEp-2	8.5	−
HEp-2 + P-1	6.1	+
HEp-2 + anti-P-1[b] 1/10	8.3	−
HEp-2 + P-1 + anti-P-1 1/10	8.3	−
HEp-2 + P-1 + anti-P-1 1/100	8.4	−
HEp-2 + P-1 + anti-P-1 1/1,000	8.2	−
HEp-2 + P-1 + anti-P-1 1/10,000	6.3	+
HEp-2	8.5	−
HEp-2 + HSV-1	10.3	+
HEp-2 + anti-HSV-1[c] 1/16	8.9	−
HEp-2 + HSV-1 + anti-HSV-1 1/16	8.8	−
HEp-2 + HSV-1 + anti-HSV-1 1/64	8.8	−
HEp-2 + HSV-1 + anti-HSV-1 1/256	9.0	−
HEp-2 + HSV-1 + anti-HSV-1 1/1,024	10.7	+

[a] = 72 h after infection; [b] = horse serum with titre 1/7,000 in neutralizing antibody; [c] = human serum with titre 1/256 in neutralizing antibody

Table 3.3   Cell water T_1 in HEp-2 cell cultures (10^6 cells) after 1 h adsorption with RSV[17]

Sample	T_1 (s)	CPE[a]
HEp-2	8.3	−
HEp-2 + RSV 10^1 PFU/cell	13.0	+
HEp-2 + RSV 10^0 PFU/cell	12.3	+
HEp-2 + RSV 10^{-1} PFU/cell	11.2	−
HEp-2 + RSV 10^{-2} PFU/cell	9.2	−
HEp-2 + RSV 10^{-3} PFU/cell	8.5	−

[a] = 30 days after infection

after 1 h of contact with permissive cells detect multiplicities of infection at least two orders of magnitude lower than the minimal one which induces a cytopathic effect (CPE). This results in a large sensitivity enhancement besides even larger time saving (1 h against 25-30 days). This feature, which is confirmed by several results, led us to suggest that the NMR measurements can detect the interaction of defective interfering virions[18], which may represent the most abundant part of a viral population, with the cell surface. The diagnostic applicability has been also tested by applying the NMR method in biological samples such as cerebrospinal fluid, stool and urine in which viruses were suspended. The sign of the change in cell water T_1, together with clinical information, may be used to speculate about the presence of a certain virus in pathological materials, although definitive identification can be performed only by virus-specific antibodies. Such identification can be suitably done by exploiting the neutralization of the NMR signal as in the case of serological diagnosis. The main problem is the availability of monospecific antisera, very reactive and not too expensive, which are not of widespread occurrence. This is just the same problem encountered in the fast-diagnosis techniques, such as ELISA, immunomicroscopy and so on. However in the case of NMR spectroscopy the advantage is that the tests utilize the antibodies having the maximum level of specificity, instead of antibodies to every viral antigen; the consequence is that the use of antisera not completely purified and unreactive against other viruses may be satisfactory.

Virological diagnosis with NMR is also possible on cell samples drawn by the infected host. The results reported in Fig. 3.3 show an easily detectable enhancement of the water T_1 in nerve cells of mice infected by fixed rabies virus when compared to healthy mice: the early detection of the NMR signal in respect of clinical symptoms, which appear 5 days later, and the direction of the T_1 change typical of enveloped viruses should be considered. Such experiments are obviously not to be extended to humans, but they represent the starting point for virological diagnosis directly on pathological material rather than by means of previous contact with permissive cells. We have gathered data concerning infection by cytomegalovirus by drawing samples of blood and urine from newborns and from their mothers. The results were promising but not completely verified, so they will not be discussed here.

The second aim of the research will be briefly exemplified by some results which, we believe, demonstrate that the evolution of the virus–cell interaction is suitably monitored by NMR spectroscopy. In cell cultures under continuous stirring the time evolution of the water T_1 in virus-infected cells and in homogeneous control cells can be studied. If the difference T_{1v} is plotted versus time (Fig. 3.4), a curve

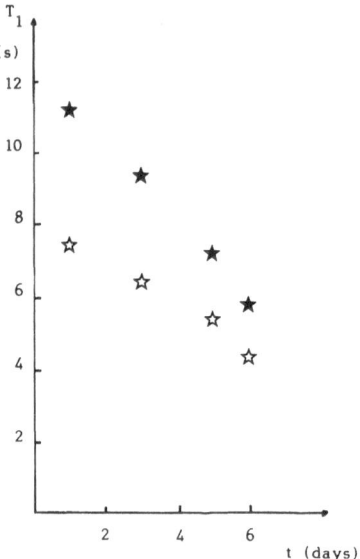

Figure 3.3   Spin–lattice relaxation times of brain water protons of healthy (white triangles) and rabies-virus infected (black triangles) mice against the time after virus infection[16]

of the cell water NMR behaviour during evolution of the virus–cell interaction is obtained. The comparison between poliovirus type 1 and vaccinia virus shows, besides the different sign and size of the NMR signal, that the two NMR signals follow the progressive steps of viral infection of a certain cell population in a completely different way. The conclusion is that a different NMR behaviour is expected for every virus–cell system. For example when persistent infection of continuously stirred HEp-2 cells by respiratory syncytial virus is induced, which is characterized by periodic production of small amounts of infectious virus from a small percentage of the cell population, the analysis of the T_{1v} curve allows a very accurate estimate of the cycles of production of infectious virus; namely, in conjunction with the cycle an abrupt change of T_{1v} is noticed, which afterward returns to normal values.

When human fetal lung diploid cells (WI-38 line) were infected by Herpes simplex virus type 2 it was possible to foretell which cell populations were going to develop productive infection just 1 h after infection. This inference, based on the cell water T_1 enhancement, was confirmed 5 days later when the cell cultures displaying a widespread

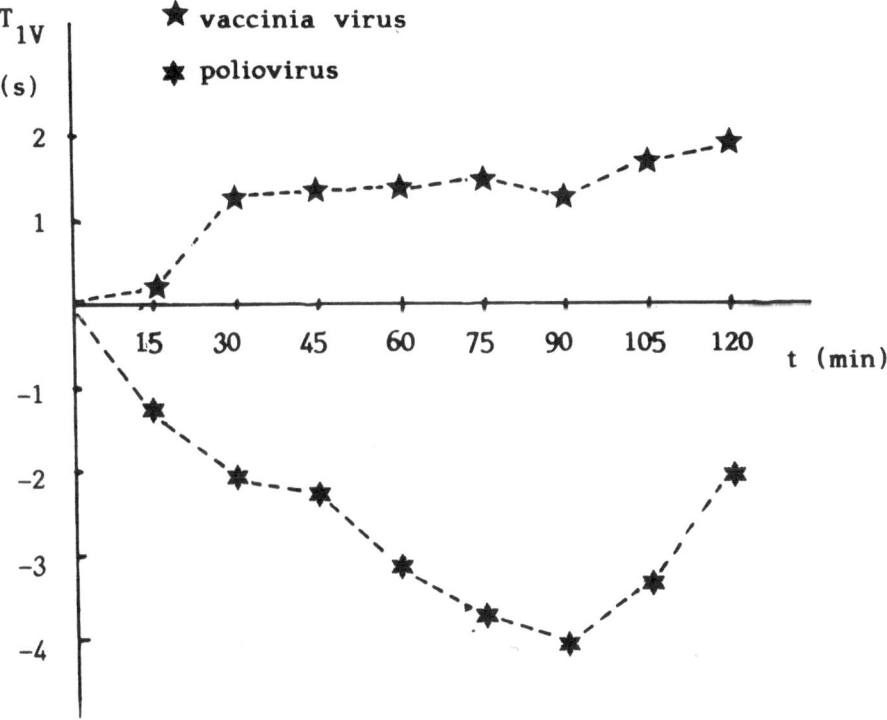

Figure 3.4 Time course of the cell water T_{1v} (see text) in growing HEp-2 cells during the early phases of the infection by poliovirus type 1 and vaccinia virus. Each sample contained 1×10^6 cells injected with 10^{-1} PFU/cell[17]

CPE showed a sharp decrease of T_1. Some of the surviving cell cultures showed, around a month later, a certain enhancement of the cell water T_1 which was the first sign of cell transformation. In fact, 40 days later we noticed the occurrence of a small number of foci of morphologically transformed cells which were then stabilized in continuous culture. All the transformed cell lines, obtained in our laboratory from WI-38 cells, display cell water T_1 values much longer than those of corresponding normal cells. Such enhancement is particularly large for the cell lines having oncogenic activity in immunosuppressed mice[19].

Using the NMR behaviour of cell water as a probe of virus-induced cell modifications requires that at least a rough knowledge of what is measured can be acquired. For this reason we run experiments with erythrocytes where the virus effect is limited to the adsorption phase. The water T_1 values in suspensions of erythrocytes are concentration-dependent and are affected by adsorption of some hemagglutinating viruses, such as Echovirus type 11 in a dose-dependent fashion. The T_1 shortening became detectable within 15 min of contact and remained constant afterwards. These findings suggest that adsorption to cell receptors is responsible, at least partially, for cell membrane modifications which result in changes in NMR properties of cell water. By making the virus adsorb suspensions of erythrocytes doped with paramagnetic Mn(II) ions or previously treated with concanavalin A and/or cytochalasin D and/or colchicine it could be inferred that the observed T_1 effect comès from modifications of the permeability properties of the cell membrane as well as from movements of the cell surface receptors closely related to the whole activity of cytoskeletal elements. Other NMR signals come from virus penetration and virus-specific macromolecular synthesis in permissive cells[20-22].

The experimental evidence collected up to now can be used to conclude that the NMR measurements are a very useful aid in studying viral infection of cells which is the first event in the evolution of many different diseases. It is our belief that the chapter of viral pathology should be largely rewritten, and that diseases linked, or somehow related, to viral vaccinations should be incorporated therein. That is why we are now extending our NMR research to cell infection by virulent wild-type viruses and by the corresponding attenuated mutants employed in preparing vaccines for humans.

REFERENCES

1. Tait, M. J. and Franks, F. (1971). Water in biological systems. *Nature*, **230**, 91–4
2. Cooke, R. and Kuntz, I. D. (1974). The properties of water in biological systems. *Ann. Rev. Biophys. Bioeng.*, **3**, 95–126
3. Hazlewood, C. F., Nichols, B. L., Chang, D. C. and Brown, B. (1974). Nuclear magnetic resonance transverse relaxation times of water protons in skeletal muscle. *Biophys. J.*, **14**, 583–606
4. Lindstrom, T. and Koenig, S. H. (1974). Magnetic-field-dependent water proton spin-lattice relaxation rates of hemoglobin solutions and whole blood. *J. Magn. Res.*, **15**, 344–53
5. Ling, G. N. and Walton, C. L. (1976). What retains water in living cells? *Science*, **191**, 293–96

6. Hollis, D. P. (1979). Nuclear magnetic resonance studies of cancer and heart disease. *Bull. Magn. Res.*, **1**, 27–37

7. Mathur-De Vrè, R. (1979). The NMR studies of water in biological systems. *Progr. Biophys. Mol. Biol.*, **35**, 103–34

8. Grosch, L. and Noack, F. (1976). NMR relaxation investigation of water mobility in aqueous bovine serum albumin solutions. *Biochim. Biophys. Acta*, **453**, 218–32

9. Edzes, H. T. and Samulski, E. T. (1977). Cross relaxation and spin diffusion in the proton NMR of hydrated collagen. *Nature*, **265**, 521–3

10. Edzes, H. T. and Samulski, E. T. (1978). The measurement of cross relaxation effects in the proton NMR spin-lattice relaxation of water in biological systems: hydrated collagen and muscle. *J. Magn. Res.*, **31**, 207–29

11. Koenig, S. H., Bryant, R. G., Hallenga, K. and Jacob, G. S. (1978). Magnetic cross-relaxation among protons in protein solutions. *Biochemistry*, **17**, 4348–58

12. Gaggelli, E., Tiezzi, E. and Valensin, G. (1979). NMR relaxation investigation of water 'ordering' in aqueous lysozyme solutions. *Chem. Phys. Lett.*, **63**, 155–8

13. Damadian, R., Zaner, K., Hor, D., Di Maio, T., Minkoff, L. and Goldsmith, M. (1973). Nuclear magnetic resonance as a new tool in cancer research: human tumors by NMR. *Ann. N.Y. Acad. Sci.*, **222**, 1048–62

14. Beall, P. T., Brinkley, B. R., Chang, D. C. and Hazlewood, C. F. (1982). Microtubule complexes correlated with growth rate and water proton relaxation times in human breast cancer cells. *Cancer Res.*, **42**, 4124–30

15. Valensin, G., Gaggelli, E., Tiezzi, E., Valensin, P. E. and Bianchi Bandinelli, M. L. (1979). The water proton spin-lattice relaxation times in virus-infected cells. *Biophys. Chem.*, **10**, 143–6

16. Valensin, P. E., Bianchi Bandinelli, M. L., Gaggelli, E., Tiezzi, E. and Valensin, G. (1980). Recognition of early virus-induced changes in cell cultures by nuclear magnetic resonance. *Microbiologica*, **3**, 25–34

17. Valensin, G., Gaggelli, E., Tiezzi, E., Valensin, P. E., Bianchi Bandinelli, M. L. and Di Cairano, M. L. (1982). Virus-cell interactions: nuclear magnetic resonance behaviour of intracellular water. *Microbiologica*, **5**, 195–205

18. Huang, A. S. (1973). Defective interfering viruses. *Ann. Rev. Microbiol.*, **27**, 101–17

19. Valensin, G., Gaggelli, E., Bianchi Bandinelli, M. L., Di Cairano, M. L. and Valensin, P. E. (1985). NMR investigations of cell cultures: early detection of infection by *Herpesvirus hominis* and of transformation. *Int. J. Cancer* (submitted)

20. Valensin, P. E., Bianchi Bandinelli, M. L., Di Cairano, M. L., Valensin, G., Gaggelli, E. and Tiezzi, E. (1981). Proton spin-lattice relaxation rates in erythrocytes adsorbed with hemagglutinating viruses. *Biophys. Chem.*, **14**, 357–62
21. Valensin, P. E., Bianchi Bandinelli, M. L., Di Cairano, M. L., Gaggelli, E. and Valensin, G. (1985). NMR parameters of local anesthetics as biological markers of the cell–virus interactions. *Arch. Virol.* **83**, 241–9
22. Valensin, G. and Valensin, P. E. (1985). Nuclear magnetic resonance probes for investigations of the virus-cell interactions. *J. Magn. Res. Med.* (in press)

4
Medical diagnosis by analytical evaluation of nuclear magnetic resonance (NMR) tomography and NMR *in vivo* spectroscopy

P. O. BRUNNER

INTRODUCTION

For some years NMR in medicine has been considered an imaging technique which is in many respects superior even to competitive techniques such as X-ray, computed tomography or ultrasound, which are widely used medical applications. Today we are ready to recognize that NMR can be a very powerful tool to learn about the complicated physical and chemical mechanisms and processes in living systems. Longitudinal and transverse relaxation of the NMR signal, as well as chemical shift data, contain structural information about tissues. Flow phenomena can be studied in connection with linear gradients to produce images, which contain pure flow information about a section of the living system. An introduction to techniques for the observation of these parameters is given in the following sections.

NMR TOMOGRAPHY AND RELAXATION TIMES

The evaluation of relaxation times always requires the development of experiments, which allow the acquisition of a representative data set within a short time. This is an intrinsic requirement for giving credence to the results, since the living system changes its state during a long sequence of experiments.

For the evaluation of the longitudinal relaxation time T_1 it is very difficult to fulfil this condition, because each measurement requires a relaxed spin system before the rf pulses are applied, to avoid partial saturation. It is therefore not possible to get real T_1 information in a single scan. The longitudinal relaxation has to be determined by several scans of the same cross-section of the body each time after the inversion pulse is varied. This is the main reason why T_1 evaluations are often based on very poor data and the values therefore contain quite high statistical errors. Nevertheless T_1 values, or at least T_1 weighted images, are very important for tissue characterization and they are in special cases significant for the diagnosis.

For the measurement of the transverse relaxation time the spin–echo technique is very well known in analytical spectroscopy. T_2 can be measured straightforwardly in one experiment, since the spin–spin relaxation starts after each perturbation of the spins by a rf pulse. For the application of the spin–echo sequence in tomography it is just as important to find an efficient imaging technique, which allows time to prepare the spins and time to recall the echoes properly. The simplest basic technique in this respect is certainly projection reconstruction, because after slice preparation no gradient switching is necessary. Whenever the slice is prepared, such that the slice spins are in field direction before the observation, the image sequence can be observed with a standard spin–echo pulse sequence and with a very short interpulse delay. The T_2 can then be evaluated with a very high accuracy due to the large number of data points which have been collected.

With the Fourier imaging technique it is also easy to perform multi-echo image sequences, but usually the interpulse delays are slightly higher because the gradients have to be switched during the observation period.

At this time, only one acquisition consisting of slice selection and observation of an echo train has been described. For the reconstruction of an image this echo-signal has to be recorded a number of times, each one in a different gradient to collect the spatial information over the sample. The reconstruction of the image itself needs only one echo of each scan. Therefore, an image data set, which consists of say 256 spatially resolving scans with 36 echoes each, can be reconstructed to 36 images of 256×256 planar volume elements. Following the intensities of a single volume element through all the 36 images, one plots an exponential function which defines T_2 with 36 data points. Depending on the interpulse delay and the specific T_2 values in the tissue, there could even be more than 36 points.

The number of data points which define the parameters is extremely important in the study of biological samples. Clearly, the accuracy of the T_2 value is very high, which means that only slightly different T_2 values in tissues can be recorded with a high certainty.

On the other hand, tissue volume elements very often contain many different chemical compounds, e.g. water and different lipids, each one with its own T_2 value. For the analysis of several T_2 values within one tissue volume element a very high number of data points is absolutely necessary.

After the evaluation of the T_2 of all the volume elements in a NMR-tomogram a virtual T_2 image can be reconstructed by the replacement of the measured intensities by the corresponding T_2. In the case of multiexponentials, overlays with the different T_2 images can be performed. The exact analysis of such a T_2 image sequence can be of very great help for medical diagnosis. Tumours surrounded by oedema very often cannot be distinguished by their signal intensities; but due to the complicated chemical structure of the tumour the multi-exponential T_2 analysis of the tumour can help to differentiate it from the oedema.

Since the method of T_2 studies by NMR tomography can be considered as very efficient, highly intensive work is required in the analysis of malignant and normal tissue in living organisms as a preparation for the later application in the medical diagnosis.

FLOW PHENOMENA IN LIVING SYSTEMS

Pathological behaviour of flow in blood vessels is a very common medical phenomenon. Its quantitative observation is difficult, however, since the characteristics of the flow are very different in the complicated system of blood vessels in a body.

Flow measurements are well known in analytical NMR. Bulk-flow along one axis has been measured to study the different characteristics and to quantify the flow either by linear flow velocity or volume flow rate.

Three main types of flow can be differentiated:

1. plug flow, which can be described by a linear flow profile;
2. laminar flow with a parabolic flow profile;

3. turbulent flow as the extreme case of plug flow at very high flow velocities.

In biological samples we have to deal most of the time with laminar flow with the addition of pulsatile excitation. The aspect of pulsed flow dramatically increases the difficulties with precise determination of flow data because in biological samples, say blood vessels, the viscosity of the blood and the elastic properties of the walls have to be included in these considerations. Problems arise also with the bends in the blood vessels, which can cause rotary motions of the fluid.

With the spatially resolving imaging technique flow effects in a biological sample can be studied in its local surroundings. In addition NMR is non-invasive and non-destructive.

Most of the techniques, which are used to determine flow effects can be included in one of the following groups:

1. time-of-flight, which describes the nuclei leaving one *rf* coil and flowing into another one;
2. inflow/outflow, the effect of inflow of fresh nuclei and the outflow of excited nuclei;
3. phase modulation of the spin–echo signal by the flowing sample in a linear field gradient.

In the last of these techniques, which can be termed the most elegant one, the phase modulation is performed by the application of a very long train of spin–echo pulses. Each odd echo of this train contains flow information due to a phase modulation, and in the even echoes the modulation effect is compensàted.

Again, the pulse sequence of the previous paragraph can be used to determine flow by spin–echo flow imaging. With this technique, flow profiles can be measured directly by the application of a read gradient in flow direction. After a slice selection and a phase encoding in one or two directions, the flow profile can be scanned as regards velocity, direction intensity and spatial distribution. The image directly represents a plot of the flow profile.

In using spin–echo flow imaging it is very straightforward to subtract the even echoes from the odd echoes to get a representation of only the flowing parts in a cross-section of the body. The possibility for the medical attendant of having flow charts of the body available will be very helpful for the diagnosis. A quantitative assignment of malignant and normal flow behaviour will be an especially powerful tool for the determination of pathological effects; but, due to the complicated structure of living systems, this field of NMR in medicine still requires many years of intensive research, as well as applications, to get experience in the interpretation of flow phenomena in the body.

IN VIVO SPECTROSCOPY

Techniques for looking at *in vivo* spectra have been developed during recent years. Surface coils are most widely used due to their high signal-to-noise ratio and easy handling. Their disadvantage with a very restricted *rf* penetration depth into the body can be avoided with a technique which enables observations of the spectrum selectively from one volume element inside the body. With a threefold selective irradiation of the sample in the x, y, z gradients respectively, a cubic volume in a region of interest can be investigated with the NMR spectrum. The experiment requires a standard imaging probe-head and therefore, due to the poor filling factor, the signal-to-noise ratio of this technique is worse than with the surface coil.

Information on a cross-section through a body with respect to spatial and chemical shift resolution can be calculated by chemical shift imaging. The information content of this method is extremely high, but it is certainly the most time-consuming one, with again a restricted signal-to-noise ratio. Very often the information is too complicated for detailed interpretation.

Although the techniques of observing *in vivo* spectra are known, this field remains, for the near future, probably the most research-oriented application of NMR in medicine. The biochemistry of the human body is very complex and the spectra, despite the signal-to-noise ratio of X-nuclei, are very often too complicated for routine application at this time.

The success of analytical high-resolution NMR has been strongly dependent on the development of highfield magnet systems. This is also certainly true for *in vivo* spectroscopy. Magnetic field strengths of 100 MHz and higher, with as large diameters as possible, will be an intrinsic requirement for basic spectroscopy work on living systems. Difficulties which arise from the individuality of each living system, can only be investigated with the help of optimum equipment.

Success in the standardization of NMR *in vivo* data will be the most important step in the direction of the routine application in medical diagnosis. Therefore the next few years in the history of *in vivo* spectroscopy will be dedicated to the collection, interpretation and standardization of spectra with the help of typical normal and malignant living samples. In most cases today research groups start work with the study of the animal organism on small NMR *in vivo* spectroscopy systems with relatively high fields of 100–200 MHz.

CONCLUSION

Due to its high information content, and because it is non-invasive and non-destructive, NMR tomography and *in vivo* spectroscopy can be much more useful for medical diagnosis than most of the competitive techniques which are already in use. But the complexity of the information, together with the individuality of the human body, requires intensive research both on tomography and *in vivo* spectroscopy. We can use these unique techniques for a better understanding of the human organism by a careful investigation of physical and biochemical parameters.

Part 2
RECOMBINANT DNA AND DNA PROBES

5
Theoretical and practical aspects of recombinant DNA techniques relevant to the clinical sciences

M. D. WINTHER

INTRODUCTION

In the past decade recombinant DNA technology has expanded out from the academic environment and into industrial and clinical laboratories around the world. Vaccines and diagnostic kits based on recombinant DNA-derived products are now available with many more practical applications soon to follow. For such products to be used effectively it is important that the potential and the limitations of the new technologies are widely understood by the whole range of specialists working in laboratory medicine. A review of the principal techniques of genetic engineering from cloning and characterizing genes to the expression of foreign antigens in *Escherichia coli*, yeast and mammalian cells will be presented. Some of the ways in which these new approaches will have a major impact on diagnosis and treatment of infections and inherited metabolic disorders will be discussed.

A few of the ways in which recombinant DNA technology will be of use to the medical sciences are listed in Table 5.1. In its primary application genetic engineering has been seen as a means of producing proteins inexpensively, but this would seem to be an excessively narrow view. Even where traditional production technologies continue to be used, recombinant DNA studies have an important contribution to make to improve the understanding of organisms and their immunologically active components. A more detailed form of quality control becomes possible where specific antigens or even

Table 5.1   Uses of recombinant DNA in the medical sciences

1.   Elucidation of the genetic basis of normal and abnormal cell function
2.   Quality control and improvement of existing biological products
3.   Alternative means of production of protein antigens currently in use in vaccines and diagnostics
4.   Production of novel protein antigens or antigens previously available in limited quantities
5.   Cloned DNA probes for the detection of the genetic material of pathogens in diagnosis

epitopes can be measured in a vaccine or diagnostic reagent. Perhaps the biggest change to affect the medical sciences in the next few years will be the introduction of cloned DNA probes for detecting pathogens or inborn errors of metabolism. This will make new demands on laboratories but the benefits will be enormous. They will also have an impact on vaccine development[1].

GENE CLONING

Recombinant DNA technology is still developing and expanding. To fully appreciate the advances that have been made it is instructive to

Table 5.2   Landmarks in the development of recombinant DNA technology

1943	Experiments by Avery, MacLeod and McCarty prove that DNA is a genetic molecule capable of altering the heredity of bacteria
1953	Watson and Crick postulate a double-helical structure for DNA
1963	Complete elucidation of the genetic code whereby a set of three nucleotides codes for a single amino acid
1970	Isolation of the first enzyme that cuts DNA molecules at specific sites, known as restriction enzymes
1972	The first *in vitro* recombinant DNA molecules generated at Stanford University utilizing DNA ligase and restriction enzymes
1978	Production of the first human hormone, somatostatin, with the use of recombinant DNA technology

review the history of this area of science. Table 5.2 lists a few of the major contributions which have come from the areas of chemistry, biochemistry and genetics. Molecular biology is a hybrid discipline, and has attracted scientists from a wide variety of backgrounds. The scientific advances came very rapidly in the 1970s with the industrial and commercial applications soon following.

Reviewed briefly, these discoveries showed that the chromosomal genetic material present in all cells consists of nucleotide sequences of deoxyribonucleic acid (DNA). These are transcribable into messenger ribonucleic acid (mRNA) and are thus directly responsible for the amino acid sequence of proteins formed in the cytoplasm of the cell. DNA normally exists within cells in a double-stranded helix with the nucleotide bases of the complementary DNA strands bound together by hydrogen bonds.

Although biochemists and geneticists recognized the importance of nucleic acids in heredity, the detailed systematic study and manipulation of DNA molecules only really became possible with the discovery of a special class of enzymes called restriction endonucleases. These enzymes recognize and cut the DNA molecule at specific sequences of nucleotides. Different restriction enzymes may recognize and cleave DNA at different places. This gives the scientist a choice of 'molecular scissors' to cut the DNA into more manageable-sized pieces.

SOURCE	ENZYME	SEQUENCE		
Escherichia coli	EcoR I	5'... G͗A A T T C	... 3'	
		3'... C T T A A͈G	... 5'	
Serratia marcescens	Sma I	5'... C C C͗G G G	... 3'	
		3'... G G G͈C C C	... 5'	
Providencia stuartii	Pst I	5'... C T G C A͗G	... 3'	
		3'... G͈A C G T C	... 5'	
Moraxella bovis	Mbo I	5'... ͗G A T C	... 3'	
		3'... C T A G͈	... 5'	

Figure 5.1 Some restriction endonuclease recognition sequences

The recognition sequences of a few restriction enzymes are given in Fig. 5.1. Over 400 different restriction enzymes have now been identified. Most restriction sites are symmetrical with the enzymes cleaving both strands of the DNA molecule. Cleavage by restriction enzymes can generate blunt ends, (as with SmaI) or 5' or 3' overhanging single-stranded ends. Note that two separate molecules that have been cut by EcoRI will have the same single-strand overhangs which are referred to as 'sticky ends'. These complementary ends can be annealed and ligated to construct a new chimeric or recombinant DNA molecule as shown in Fig. 5.2.

The essential feature of recombinant DNA technology is that it enables one to construct new DNA molecules *in vitro* and to specifically transfer genetic information from one organism into another. The initial cloning experiments used the bacteria *E. coli* as the recipient

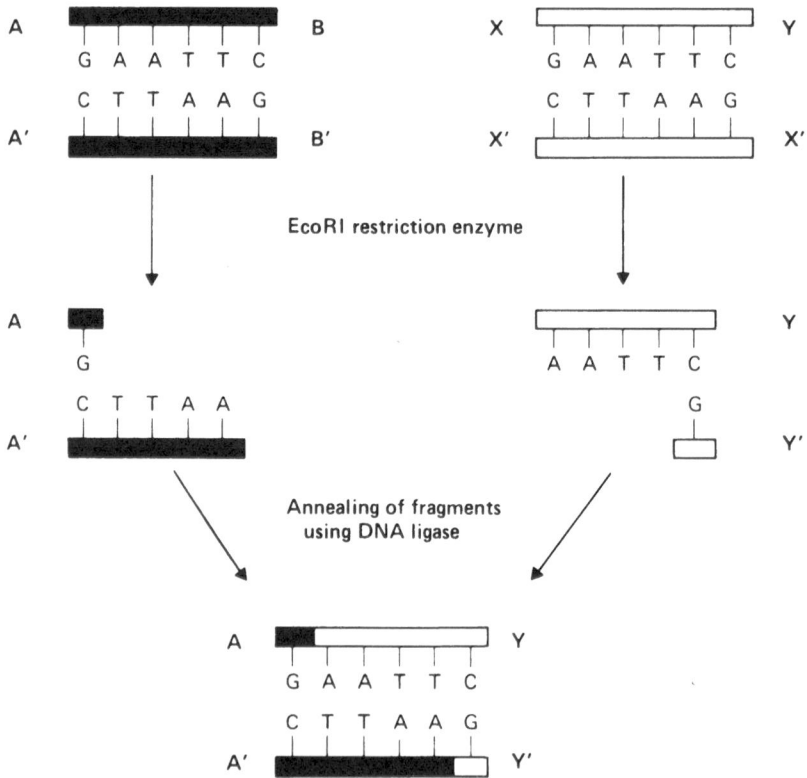

Figure 5.2   Cutting and ligation of DNA fragments

for the chimeric molecules, but it is now possible to transfer DNA into a wide range of bacteria, yeast, plant cells and mammalian cells. A variety of specialized vectors have been developed which can be used for cloning experiments which have greatly increased the power and scope of this new technology.

The principles of genetic engineering are most easily illustrated with bacteria such as *E. coli* (Fig. 5.3). The bulk of the genetic information in the cell is contained in a single circular chromosome of about 4 million base pairs length. This is sufficient to code for several thousand average-sized proteins. Many bacteria also contain additional genetic elements known as plasmids, which can be from only a few thousand to over 50 000 base pairs in size. Plasmids code for only a few proteins which specify essential plasmid replication functions and frequently auxiliary functions which enhance the host's viability or

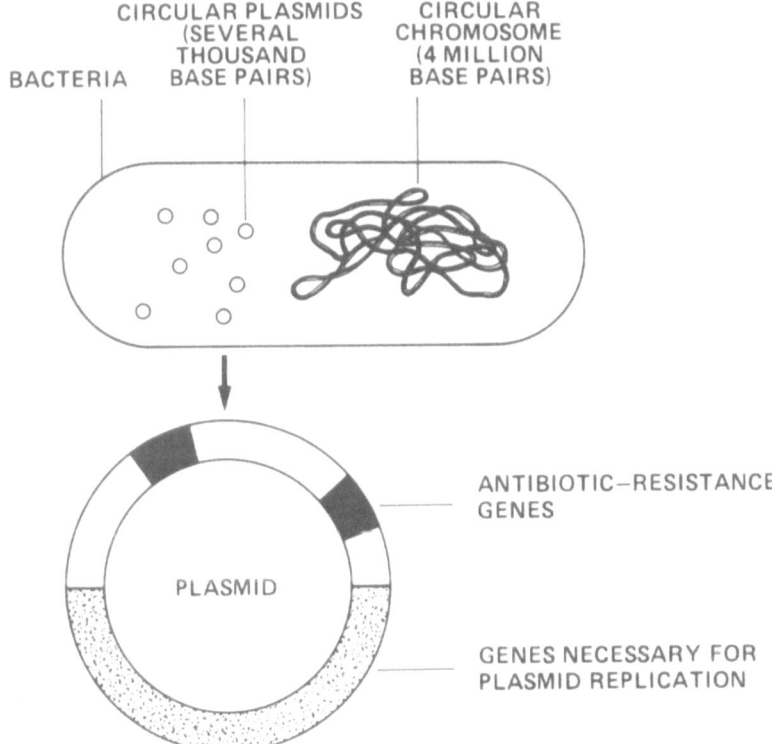

Figure 5.3   Bacterial plasmids

pathogenicity. Many genes for antibiotic resistance, heavy metal resistance or other virulence factors are contained on plasmids. Plasmids can be present in low copy numbers (1 or 2 per cell) or in high copy numbers (30 or more per cell), depending on the nature of the replication control.

The most commonly used plasmid, pBR322, has been completely characterized at the nucleotide level. This circular double-stranded DNA plasmid of 4363 base pairs carries the genes for ampicillin and tetracycline resistance in addition to its replication functions. Foreign DNA can be cloned into various parts of this plasmid without affecting its replication functions. The process of cloning foreign DNA in a plasmid is summarized in Fig. 5.4. After the recombinant DNA molecule is introduced into the host cell, the transformed cells are selected from the non-transformed cells by virtue of the antibiotic resistance gene located on the plasmid.

A 'gene bank' can be constructed for an organism by cloning all of its chromosomal DNA onto plasmids in *E. coli*. A gene bank for a bacteria (average genome size $= 4 \times 10^6$ base pairs) would require several thousand different recombinant clones with pBR322 as the vector. Using a specially modified form of plasmid, known as a cosmid, much larger pieces of DNA may be cloned such that a collection of 200 cosmids can represent an entire bacterial genome. Mammalian genomes are considerably larger and a cosmid bank of 10^5–10^6 separate clones would be required.

Due to the very large numbers of clones that need to be generated and examined with large genomes, it may be preferable to make gene banks only from the actively expressed genes. For this purpose a process called cDNA cloning is used[2]. This involves the enzymatic conversion of polyadenylated messenger RNA into double-stranded DNA and subsequent insertion into a bacterial plasmid (Fig. 5.5).

Having generated genomic of cDNA gene banks, it is necessary to identify the individual clone coding for the protein you are interested in. This can be the most difficult step for some genes. There are two basic approaches to identifying a clone. (1) Where specific high-titre antisera is available, immunological techniques are possible. The success of this depends on achieving some expression of the foreign gene in the host. (2) Where partial amino acid sequences of the protein are known it is possible to synthesize the corresponding oligonucleotide DNA sequence(s) and to carry out DNA hybridization experiments. Only the bacterial colony containing the desired gene will

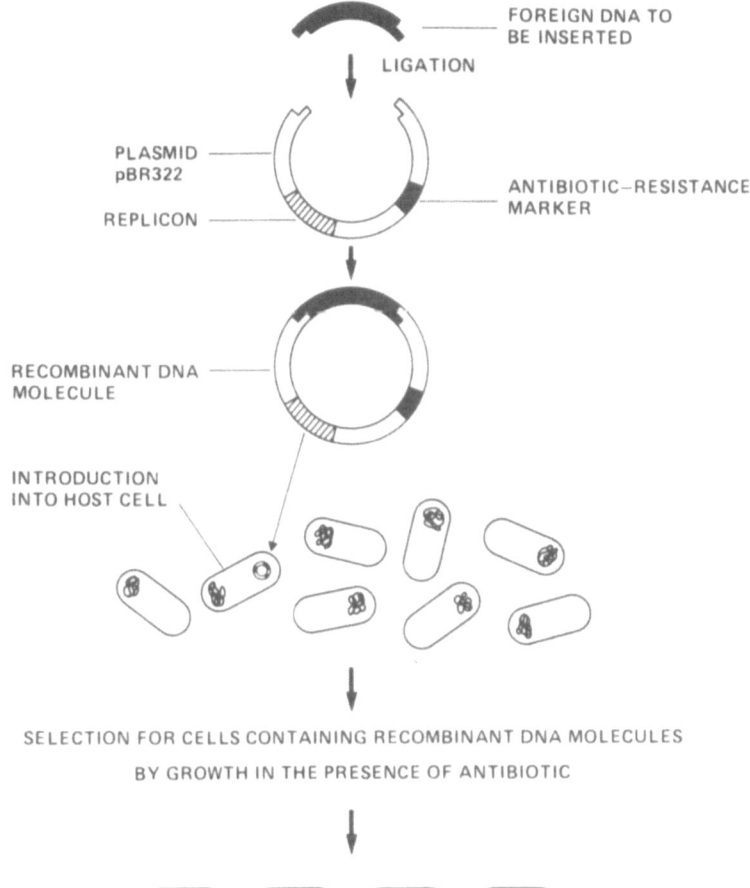

FOREIGN DNA TO
BE INSERTED

LIGATION

PLASMID
pBR322

ANTIBIOTIC–RESISTANCE
MARKER

REPLICON

RECOMBINANT DNA
MOLECULE

INTRODUCTION
INTO HOST CELL

SELECTION FOR CELLS CONTAINING RECOMBINANT DNA MOLECULES
BY GROWTH IN THE PRESENCE OF ANTIBIOTIC

Figure 5.4   Cloning DNA in a plasmid

hybridize to the synthetic probe. Unfortunately the 'degeneracy' of the genetic code, by which a single amino acid may be coded for by several different triplet codons, means that a large number of sequences are possible and a complex oligonucleotide mixture needs to be synthesized.

For small proteins whose complete amino acid sequence is known, it is also possible to chemically synthesize the entire gene. This approach has been used for small peptide hormones and interferon.

Having obtained a clone of the desired gene the next step is to determine its structure and properties on a molecular level. Here the

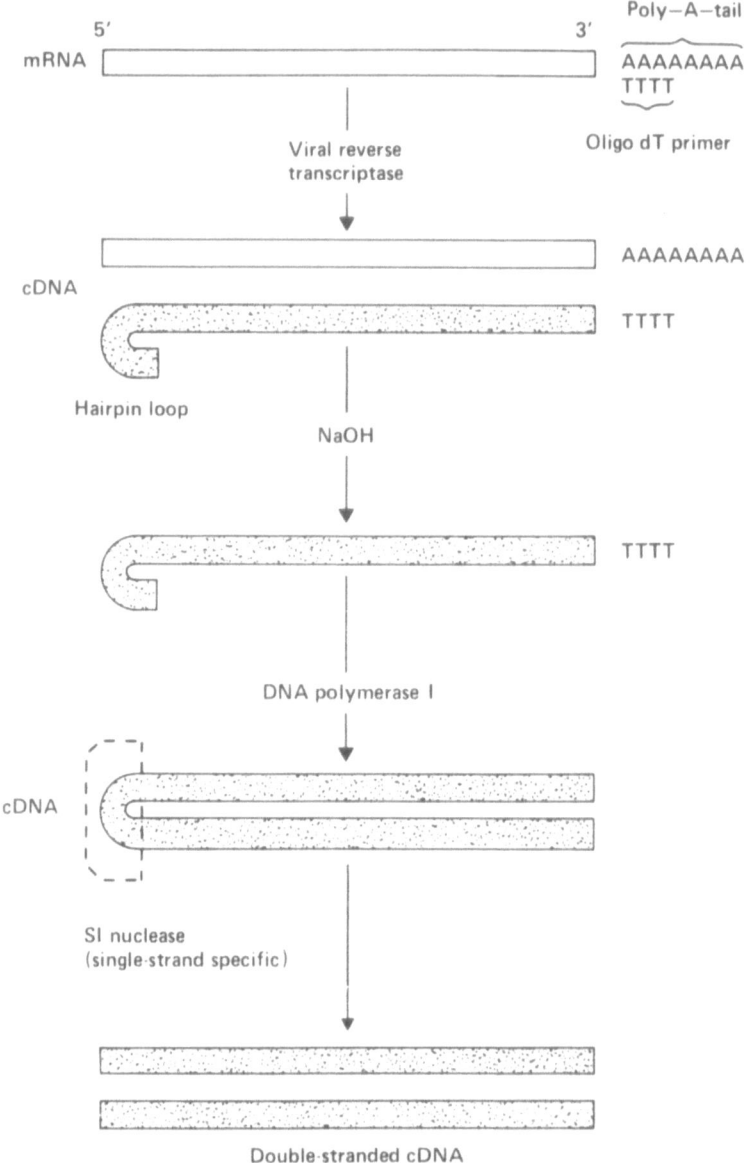

Figure 5.5 Synthesis of double-stranded cDNA

breakthrough came with the development of techniques which allow one to determine the exact nucleotide sequence of the cloned insert[3,4]. Knowledge of the nucleotide sequences allows one to predict the amino acid sequence of the encoded protein if this is not already known. This is particularly important where the protein is not available in sufficient quantities to allow the amino acid sequence to be determined by chemical techniques.

GENE EXPRESSION

Where the goal of genetic engineering is to produce proteins in *E. coli* then it is usually necessary to carry out a number of alterations to the originally cloned gene to enable high levels of expression to occur. The gene will need to be precisely modified and inserted into expression vector[5, 6]. Expression vectors contain sequences of DNA that are required for the efficient transcription of their mRNAs in *E. coli*. Such vectors are essential for expressing eukaryotic genes in *E. coli* but are also useful for increasing production of prokaryotic gene products. Although the vast majority of expression vectors are plasmid-based there are now examples of the use of bacteriophage expression vectors as well[7].

To achieve high levels of expression the foreign gene must be placed under the control of an *E. coli* promoter that is efficiently recognized by RNA polymerase. Eukaryotic promoters have no activity in bacteria so bacterial regulatory sequences must be used. The mRNA that is synthesized must also have further sequences to allow ribosomes to bind at the correct place to initiate translation. The protein that results must be stable and not subject to proteolytic degradation if high levels of accumulation are to occur.

Although the techniques for optimizing the expression of genes in *E. coli* are quite advanced – with foreign proteins being made at up to 20% of total cell protein – some proteins are difficult to produce in this way and alternative hosts may be required. For example, hepatitis B surface antigen is expressed poorly in *E. coli* but at high levels in the yeast, *Saccharomyces cerevisiae*[8]. Mammalian cells as hosts for this kind of work have the further advantage of carrying out post-translational modifications such as glycosylation which may be important for producing biologically active molecules.

SUMMARY

The ability to construct chimeric molecules and move genetic determinants between species has opened up new approaches to vaccine and diagnostics development. This has now developed into an exciting area of research which requires multidisciplinary teams to solve problems of protein structure and confirmation, microbial pathogenicity and the immune system. Recombinant DNA techniques are useful both as a tool of analysis and as a means of antigen production. Although many new vaccines are likely to result from the new technologies, there are few new products on the market at this time. This shows that the production of totally new vaccines is more difficult than expected. The ultimate success of the new products rests on consumer acceptance and costs. Recombinant DNA technology must be fully integrated into the more traditional pharmaceutical practices to accomplish this final goal.

REFERENCES

1. Winther, M. D. and Dougan, G. (1984). The impact of new technologies on vaccine development. *Biotechnol. Genet. Eng. Rev.*, **2**, 1–39
2. Williams, J. G. (1981). The preparation and screening of a cDNA clone bank. In Williamson, R. (ed.) *Genetic Engineering*. Vol. 1, pp. 1–59. (New York: Academic Press)
3. Maxam, A. M. and Gilbert, W. (1977). A new method for sequencing DNA. *PNAS*, **74**, 560–4
4. Sanger, F., Nicklen, S. and Coulson, A. R. (1977). DNA sequencing with chain terminating inhibitors. *PNAS*, **74**, 5463–7
5. Roberts, T. M. and Lauer, G. D. (1979). Maximizing gene expression on a plasmid using recombination *in vitro*. *Methods Enzymol.*, **68**, 473–81
6. Guarante, L., Roberts, T. M. and Ptashne, M. (1980). A technique for expressing eukaryotic genes in bacteria. *Science*, **209**, 1428–30
7. Young, R. A. and Davis, R. W. (1983). Efficient isolation of genes by using antibody probes. *PNAS*, **80**, 1194–8
8. Valenzuela, P., Medina, A., Rutter, W. J., Ammerer, G. and Hall, B. D. (1982). Synthesis and assembly of hepatitis B virus surface antigen particles in yeast. *Nature*, **298**, 347–50

6
The use of gene manipulation for the production of antigens

P. E. HIGHFIELD

INTRODUCTION

There are a number of advantages associated with genetically engineered material:

1. no necessity to handle infected and possibly infectious material;
2. no necessity to culture difficult to handle organisms;
3. can obtain the antigen of interest free from other antigens of the organism;
4. high yields are possible;
5. chimeric antigen–enzyme fusions possible.

Because of these advantages, genetic engineering may lead to the development of some new diagnostic tests by providing relatively large amounts of pure, specific antigens.

NEW TECHNIQUES

The stages of development in expression of a foreign antigen are:

1. *Obtain DNA coding for the antigen of interest, e.g. cDNA, genome DNA, synthetic DNA*

It is obviously necessary to have cloned DNA. However, for many eukaryotic genes it is not possible to use genomic DNA for expression in bacteria. The coding sequences of some eukaryotic genes can be found as coding regions (exons) separated by non-coding regions (introns); the bacterial cell cannot properly express such genes. There-fore it is necessary to use intron-less DNA where the coding sequences are contiguous, e.g. cDNA.

2. Determine the sequence of DNA
This step is not essential but subsequent manipulations of the DNA are much easier to plan and execute when some sequence data are available. Modern techniques of sequencing enable quite large pieces of DNA to be analysed quickly.

3. Modify the DNA to facilitate the addition of control sequences
Foreign genes need bacterial control sequences before they can be expressed. These control sequences include promoter/operator regions, ribosome binding sites and translational initiation sites. The foreign gene will need to be modified so that these sequences can be conveniently introduced. It is at this point that the expression strategy can be decided upon. The particular bacterial control elements to be introduced are chosen and a suitable protocol planned.

4. Construct plasmid designed for expression
This is not a restatement of the previous stage, but emphasizes that it is often most convenient to carry out some manipulations in a non-expressing vector background. When the foreign gene has been suitably modified it can be transferred into an expression plasmid. In some cases expression of foreign proteins can be detrimental to the bacteria and so will be selected against. It is best therefore to leave this potential complication to the final stages of the construction.

5. Assay of expression
Even the best-planned expression constructions may not give the expected levels of antigen, or the antigen may have altered properties. Some polypeptides are very unstable when expressed in bacteria and do not accumulate.

6. Modify the constructions as necessary to improve expression
The constructions can be modified either drastically, by introducing different controlling sequences, or subtly, by minor sequence changes, to maximize expression. Whilst the basic ground-rules for expression are known, and certain promoters and ribosome binding sites have been identified as giving good levels of expression, the introduction of foreign gene sequences next to them can have an unpredictable effect on their functioning. So it may be necessary to replace one

controlling element with another or alter the sequences around the gene to increase expression.

By way of illustration this approach has been applied to expressing HBcAg in *E. coli*. HBcAg is associated with the particulate structure surrounding the HBV DNA in the virion and this core particle consists of multiple copies of one polypeptide which is encoded by the core gene. Another important antigen, HBeAg, can be derived from the core antigen by disrupting this core particle. So the product of the core gene can give rise to two important HBV antigens: HBcAg and HBeAg. Antibodies against these antigens are important markers of viral infection and subsequent clearance. Presently HBcAg is isolated from infected human liver at low yield (1 µg/g of tissue) and HBeAg is only obtainable from infectious serum, which gives problems for large-scale production.

The virus has a DNA genome and can be cloned into plasmids. One such plasmid (pHB3) has been modified to introduce a BamHI site 100 bp upstream of the core gene. It was decided to fuse the core gene onto the trpE gene of *E. coli* which is under the control of the trypto-phan operon promoter (Ptrp); fusions of this type have previously given high levels of expression. The trpE gene was modified by intro-ducing a BamHI site about 150 bp within the gene and the two modified genes were brought together on one plasmid (pWRL3100). The two genes were fused randomly following exonuclease digestion around the unique BamHI site. Colonies containing fused genes were screened immunologically for expression of core antigen. Positive colonies were used to prepare cell-free extracts which could be tested in liquid assays and the core antigen quantitated. Table 6.1 shows the results of a number of assays on some of the clones and the best expression obtained was 30 mg core/l/E600 for clone 3127; this is equivalent to a total of 80 mg from 1 l of culture. In the electron microscope the core antigen could be seen as 27 nm particles which were identical in appearance to core particles obtained from infected livers. Further-more, these core particles can be disaggregated giving rise to HBeAg.

So genetic engineering techniques have allowed us to produce large amounts of two important HBV antigens free from any infectious material. The core antigen accounts for a small percentage of the total bacterial protein and can be fairly easily purified; however purifi-cation may not be necessary for its use as a diagnostic reagent. The bacterially produced HBcAg and eAg have performed well in diag-nostic tests for anti-core or anti-e antibodies.

Table 6.1

	Expt I +IA	Expt II +TRP	+IA	Expt III +IA	Expt IV +IA	Expt V +IA
3123	—	0.1*	9			
3125	—	ND	0.2			
3127	—	0.2	10	5	6	30
3129	—	ND	0.3			
3131	10	—	—	10	12.5	
3132	5	—	—			
3149	2	—	—			

* MG core/l/E600; ND not detectable

OUTLOOK

Genetic engineering can be used to produce antigens in bacteria. This development is of particular importance when antigens are required to assess the immunological response to an infection or other diseased condition, particularly when they are difficult to obtain by conventional techniques.

7
DNA probes in microbiology

G. DOUGAN

INTRODUCTION

The successful diagnosis of a microbial infection is dependent on the ability to confirm the presence of material from pathogenic micro-organisms in clinical samples. The diagnostic approaches will vary according to the clinical situation but any test must be able to identify a potential pathogen, or material from that pathogen, amongst complex biological material. In order to identify a particular micro-organism it is necessary to take advantage of special characteristics which are unique or commonly associated with that micro-organism. In addition, to be clinically and commercially successful, tests should in general be reliable, economic and easy to perform by trained personnel. A variety of approaches have been used routinely to identify infectious agents in the clinical diagnostics laboratory. Simple bacteriological techniques including cultivation of samples on selective or differential growth media and biotyping have been in successful use for decades. These approaches take advantage of particular metabolic traits associated with individual pathogens. Since specificity is one of the main requirements of a diagnostic reagent, immunological techniques have proved to be of immense value. Indeed, most of the recently developed diagnostic kits employ antibodies which bind specifically to particular bacterial or viral associated antigens. Since all micro-organisms possess unique as well as cross-reactive antigens, an immunological approach can be used at some stage in their identification.

As well as possessing species-specific antigens all species of micro-organisms contain portions of their genetic material which are unique to that micro-organism. Thus, if a simple and sensitive technique was available for the identification of unique 'genes' amongst a mixture of genomes from different organisms, this could provide the basis for a rational alternative approach to the diagnosis of microbial infections.

The genetic material present in all cells consists of the nucleic acid, deoxyribonucleic acid (DNA), although some viruses have genomes consisting of ribonucleic acid (RNA). DNA normally exists within cells in a double-stranded form with the nucleotide bases of the complementary DNA strands bound together by hydrogen bonds. The sequence and organization of the nucleotide bases within the DNA (or RNA) of the genome, determines the genetic structure of the organism.

Although common nucleotide sequences can be shared between the genomes of different organisms, all species have DNA or RNA sequences which are unique to that organism. Under appropriate conditions a single-stranded form of a particular nucleotide sequence can only bind to the corresponding complementary sequence, even if a complex mixture of other DNA sequences is present. Thus a single-stranded DNA fragment from a unique portion of a micro-organism's genome would bind to its complementary strand present in the genome of the organism from which it originated and not to the genomes of any other organism which might be present in a clinical or biological sample. If large quantities of a DNA fragment encoding a unique nucleotide sequence from an individual pathogen were purified and labelled or 'tagged' in some way to distinguish it from other DNA molecules, it could be used as a probe to detect the presence of complementary sequences within complex DNA mixtures or properly prepared biological samples. The technology to carry out this approach at the research laboratory level has been available for several years and it is now being adapted so that it can be applied practically in the diagnostics laboratory.

The first really successful development of the use of DNA fragments to probe mixtures of DNA molecules for the presence of complementary sequences was provided by Southern[1]. This technique is commonly referred to as 'Southern blotting'. In his original paper, Southern employed the use of purified target DNA fractionated electrophoretically on agarose gels. However, the technique can be adapted for use with impure DNA prepared directly from bacterial colonies or clinical samples, although in such cases non-specific background reactions can occur due to the presence of all material other than DNA, e.g. proteins. Gene cloning as a means of generating probes has already been described in a previous chapter[2].

In either procedure a DNA or RNA fragment encoding a particular nucleotide sequence to be used as a probe is purified free from contaminating biological material and other DNA fragments. The probe is then radioactively labelled to high specific activity by incorporating [32]P- or ^{35}S-labelled nucleotides *in vitro* into the DNA in a reaction involving the use of DNA polymerases, known as 'nick-translation'. Thus ^{32}P or ^{35}S is incorporated directly into the probe and any unincorporated nucleotides are removed. The radiolabelled DNA is then denatured to a single-stranded form and mixed under carefully controlled hybridization conditions with target DNA (see Fig. 7.1). The target DNA is normally bound prior to hybridization to a solid matrix such as nitrocellulose paper. The matrix-bound target DNA and labelled probe are incubated under conditions which favour binding of the probe *only* to its complementary strand. Thus the probe will not bind to samples which do not contain the complementary sequence. Following incubation the solid matrix is washed under conditions which remove non-specifically bound probes, and specifically bound probes can be identified following autoradiography or counting.

RADIOACTIVE
PROBE
[32]P, [35]S

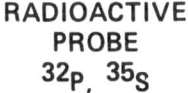
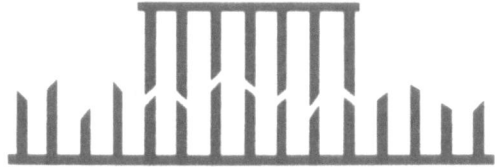

DNA template

Figure 7.1 Radioactive probe

GENOME-SPECIFIC PROBES

In order to be useful as a diagnostic tool a probe must be specific for the genome of an individual or well-characterized group of pathogens. Total chromosomal DNA prepared from any micro-organism is a complex mixture of DNA sequences some of which are likely to cross-hybridize to DNA from other species. Thus this is not suitable for use as a specific probe. Two approaches, both employing gene cloning, can be used to prepare species-specific probes. In the first approach DNA fragments representative of the total genomic DNA of a pathogen can be cloned using the *Escherichia coli* K12 host/vector system. DNA fragments from individual recombinants are then purified, labelled and used to probe DNA from the parental organism and DNA from a wide range of other species. DNA fragments which only hybridize to DNA from the parental organism can be selected for use as specific probes. The second approach involves the cloning in *E. coli* K12 of genetic determinants known to be associated with particular pathogens. Examples include the genes for the toxin of the *Corynebacterium diphtheriae* or α-toxin of *Staphylococcus aureus*. DNA encoding the cloned gene is then tested for specificity as a probe. Both approaches have been used to identify specific probes and now a large number are available for micro-organisms including *Neisseria gonorrhoeae*, chlamydiae and hepatitis B virus.

APPLICATION OF DNA PROBES TO EPIDEMIOLOGICAL STUDIES AND DIAGNOSIS OF INFECTIOUS DISEASE

A number of attempts have been made to develop the use of DNA probes in diagnosis. Pioneering work carried out by workers in Stanley Falkow's laboratory can serve as an illustrative example of the approaches taken[3]. Enterotoxigenic strains of *E. coli* (ETEC) are recognized as a major cause of diarrhoea in humans. One impediment to the diagnosis of these infections has been the difficulty in distinguishing ETEC from the *E. coli* present in the normal flora. ETEC produce two distinct classes of enterotoxin, known as the heat-labile (LT) or heat-stable (ST) toxins. Up until recently the only assays for the detection of enterotoxin-producing organisms involved the use of animals or tissue culture techniques, although immunological assays have now been developed. Falkow's group used gene cloning techniques to identify and prepare DNA fragments encoding either the LT or ST toxins, and showed that these fragments could be used in the laboratory as specific probes for ETEC. Field work was then carried out using patients suffering from diarrhoea in Bangladesh. The toxin probes were used to detect *E. coli* colonies grown and lysed *in situ* on nitrocellulose filters, and also to detect the presence of ETEC in bacterial growth in directly spotted stools from patients with acute diarrhoea. The probe technique showed a high correlation with other methods for detecting ETEC.

Falkow and other workers have extended these types of studies to the diagnosis of other infections including gonorrhoea. However, although the assay is sensitive, detecting nanogram quantities of DNA and as few as 100 micro-organisms in a clinical sample, the uses of ^{32}P label is not acceptable in routine diagnostic assays, and thus alternative labels for DNA are required if the technique is to gain general acceptance.

NON-RADIOACTIVE DNA LABELLING

Intensive efforts have been made to develop alternative methods for labelling DNA probes. One of the most successful approaches has been the development of so called 'Biotin-labelled probes' (Fig. 7.2). Biotin (vitamin A) can be bound to avidin, a glycoprotein, with extremely high affinity (Kd of 10^{-15} mol/l). Biotin can also be incorporated into DNA in the form of a dTTp or dUTP analogue using the nick-translation reaction. The incorporation of biotin into DNA does not greatly affect its ability to bind to complementary strands. The resulting biotinated probe has the advantage of being relatively stable

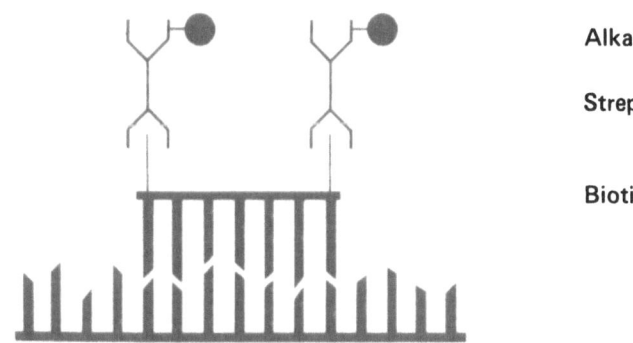

Alkaline phosphatase

Streptavidin

Biotinylated probe

Figure 7.2   Biotin probe

and non-radioactive. The detection of biotinated probes involves the formation of biotin–avidin complexes which are then picked up by conventional ELISA or fluorescent antibody techniques incorporating the use of coupled avidin or anti-avidin antibodies[4]. The technique has been developed to the extent that viral DNA can be readily detected in cultured cells or paraffin-embedded infected tissue section samples[5].

FUTURE DEVELOPMENTS

A number of laboratories are specializing in the development of diagnostic kits based on the use of DNA probes and biotinated reagents. It remains to be seen how acceptable the kits become for routine use and how they will compare with conventional immunological approaches. One proposed major use of DNA probes is in the routine screening for Salmonellae.

REFERENCES

1. Southern, E. M. (1975). Detection of specific sequences among DNA fragments separated by electrophoresis. *J. Mol. Biol.*, **98**, 503–17
2. Winther, M. D. (1985). In Shinton, N. K. (ed.) *New Technologies in Clinical Laboratory Science*. pp. 35–44. (Lancaster: MTP Press)
3. Moseley, S. L., Huq, I., Alim, A. R. M. A., So, M., Samadpour-Motalebi, M. and Falkow, S. (1980). Detection of enterotoxigenic *Escherichia coli* by DNA colony hybridisation. *J. Infect. Dis.*, **142**, 892–8
4. Leary, J., Brigati, D. J. and Ward, D. C. (1983). Rapid and sensitive colorimetric method for visualising biotin-labeled DNA probes hybridised to DNA or RNA immobilized on nitrocellulose. Bio-blots. *Proc. Natl. Acad. Sci. USA*, **80**, 4045–9
5. Brigati, D. J., Myerson, D., Leary, J. J., Spalholz, B., Travis, S. Z., Fong, C. K. Y., Hsiung, G. D. and Ward, D. C. (1983). Detection of viral genomes in cultured cells and paraffin-embedded tissue sections using biotin-labeled hybridisation probes. *Virology*, **126**, 32–50.

8
The use of DNA probes in the prenatal diagnosis of inherited metabolic disorders

F. GÜTTLER

INTRODUCTION

The human genomic DNA is constructed of approximately 3 billion nucleotides in specific sequences forming very long molecules. These DNA sequences (exons) are the chromosomal material bearing the genetic information of living cells. The coding DNA sequences of the gene are interrupted by non-coding intervening sequences or introns (see Fig. 8.1).

Recent advances in recombinant DNA technology, including restriction endonuclease analysis, has provided a wealth of information about human molecular pathology. Restriction endonuclease analysis of DNA is increasingly used as a tool for carrier detection and prenatal diagnosis of genetic disorders for which there was so far no available methodology. This is possible in the early fetus, because the DNA defect is present in every cell, including cultured fibroblasts, amniotic fluid cells, and chorionic villi trophoblasts[1,2].

In order to diagnose a genetic disease by DNA analysis, the abnormal gene must be found by using gene *probes*[3] (Fig. 8.1) and *restriction endonucleases* (Fig. 8.3) that cleave DNA at predictable sites[4]. The fragments of total human DNA digests produced by these enzymes can be separated according to their size in agarose gels (Fig. 8.4). The position of the particular gene or gene fragments among thousands of others can be determined by *hybridization* (Fig. 8.2) with a labelled gene probe followed by autoradiography (Fig. 8.4). The hybridization reaction is highly specific and occurs only between *complementary* lengths of DNA (Fig. 8.2). By means of reverse transcriptases, mRNA can be used as template to make an exactly complementary DNA

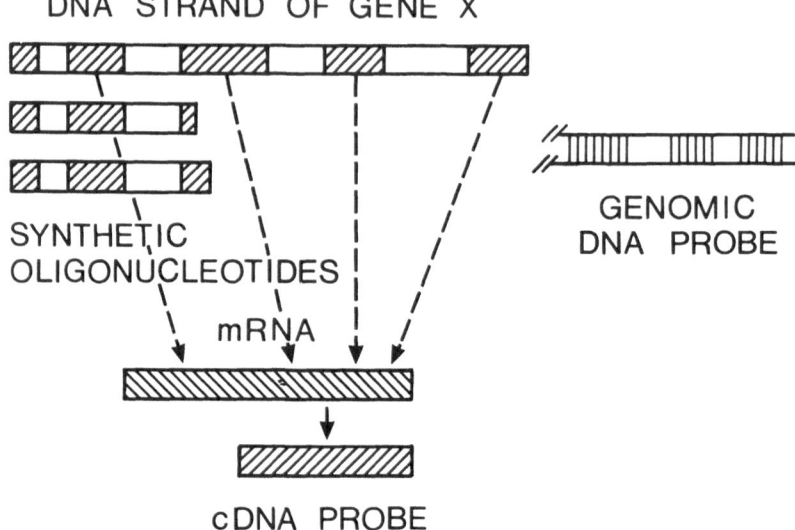

Figure 8.1 The DNA strands of gene X and the corresponding types of probes: synthetic oligonucleotides, a genomic DNA probe and a complementary DNA or cDNA probe. ▨exon; ☐intron; ▧complementary nucleotide sequence; mRNA, messenger RNA

Complementary sequences

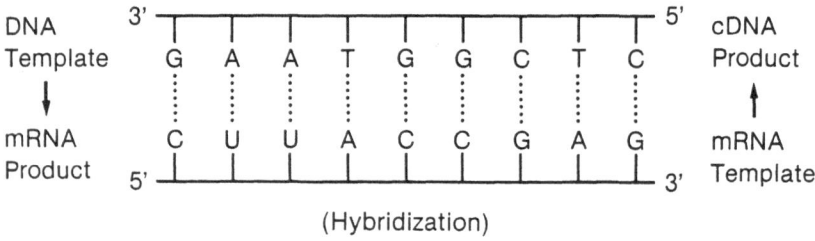

(Hybridization)

Figure 8.2 The complementary relationship between messenger RNA (mRNA) product and DNA template, as well as the relationship between mRNA template and cDNA product, is illustrated. RNA polymerase takes instructions from the DNA template strand to synthesize the mRNA nucleotide sequence which is exactly complementary to that of the DNA template strand. Reverse transcriptase takes instructions from the nucleotide sequence of mRNA to synthesize the exactly complementary nucleotide sequences of the cDNA probe. Only complementary nucleotide sequences of DNA will hybridize during the hybridization reaction described in Fig. 8.4 (1)

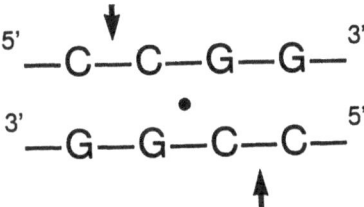

Figure 8.3 The recognition sequence of the restriction endonuclease *Msp*I. Arrows indicate the sites of cleavage

(cDNA) probe (Figs. 8.1 and 8.2) which can be used to search the genome for its partner.

Recent advances in the study of human DNA suggests that any one individual has a variant but inherited nucleotide for every 100–300 of the 3 billion nucleotides in the genome. These nucleotide variations are responsible for the presence or absence of recognition sites for restriction endonucleases (Fig. 8.3). The result is individual variations in the size of some of the DNA fragments obtained after digestion with a restriction endonuclease and a unique pattern of DNA fragments is obtained.

The presence and absence of the restriction endonuclease sites are harmless structural variations in the introns that are inherited in a simple Mendelian fashion. Hence, by use of a battery of restriction enzymes and a radioactive cDNA probe (Fig. 8.4) different lengthened fragments of DNA will appear according to the presence or absence of these polymorphic sites. Such restriction fragment length polymorphisms (RFLPs) provide a source of genetic markers that can be used to trace mutant genes to which they are linked through successive generations of families.

The experimental procedure for detection of genes by restriction endonuclease analysis of chromosomal DNA (Fig. 8.4)

Genomic DNA is isolated from fibroblasts, leucocytes, amniotic fluid cells or chorionic villi trophoblasts. DNA is cut by a restriction enzyme (Fig. 8.4 (1)) into a million or so fragments of discrete length depending on the recognition sequences that are present at the DNA molecule of the individual and the particular restriction enzyme that has been used.

The DNA fragments are separated according to size by electrophoresis in an agarose gel (Fig. 8.4 (2)). After the electrophoresis the DNA fragments can be visualized by staining with ethidium bromide

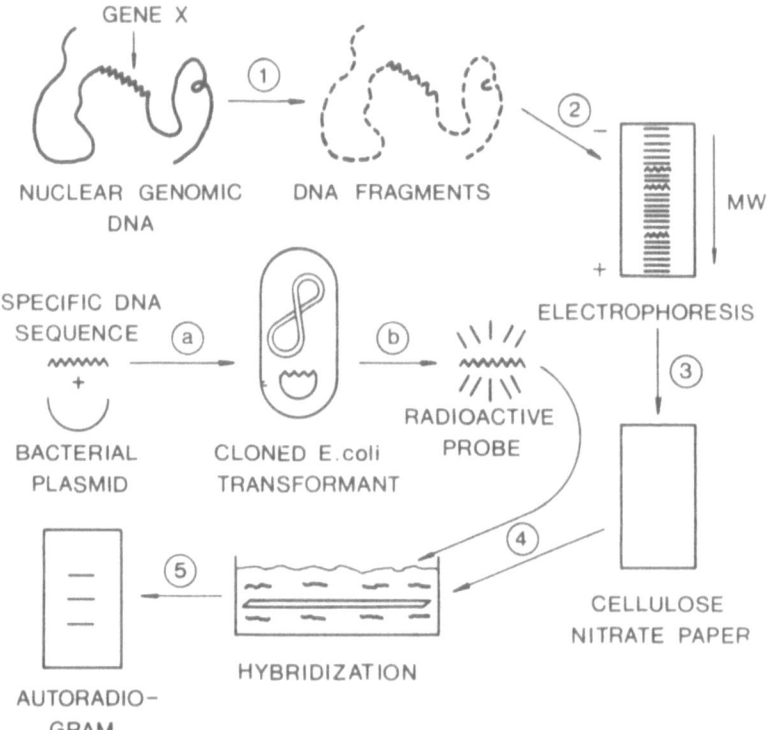

Figure 8.4   Steps in restriction endonuclease analysis of DNA. (1) Restriction endonuclease digestion. (2) Separation according to size. (3) Blot-transfer. (a) DNA complementary in sequence to gene X is inserted into a bacterial plasmid and cloned. (b) The specific DNA sequence is isolated from the recombinant plasmid and serves as the gene probe. (4) The radioactive probe will find and hybridize with homologous DNA gene fragments. (5) Restriction fragments containing gene X sequences appear as bands on the developed film

and examination of the gel in UV light. The DNA fragments in the gel can be transferred onto a piece of nitrocellulose filter (Fig. 8.4 (3)) and the filter challenged with a specific hybridization probe (Fig. 8.4 (4)) labelled with 32-phosphorus (Fig. 8.4 (b)). The labelled DNA probe will recognize its complementary counterpart on the filter (cf. Fig. 8.2) and the probe will be retained specifically, i.e. hybridize with homologous DNA fragments (Fig. 8.4 (4)). After hybridization the filter is washed to remove unhybridized radioactivity and subjected to auto-radiography. Using these methods, DNA fragments which have hybridized with the radioactive probe appear as bands on the developed film (Fig. 8.4 (5)).

Tracing mutant genes in linkage analysis using cloned complementary (cDNA) gene probes revealing DNA polymorphisms

Purified mRNA can be used to construct a complementary cDNA sequence (Fig. 8.1 and Table 8.1) which is then used to screen a human liver cDNA library. During these experiments a cDNA clone (Fig. 8.4 (b)) can be isolated, which reveals restriction fragment length polymorphisms (RFLPs). When RFLPs have been established the probe can then be used to detect the corresponding gene in the human genome of families suffering from a genetic disorder. Thus the technique can be applied for prenatal diagnosis and carrier detection of inherited disorders (Table 8.1).

Table 8.1 Examples of genetic disorders which can be analysed using complementary cDNA gene probes to detect closely linked polymorphisms

Disease	Probes
Antithrombin III deficiency	cDNA (antithrombin III)
Growth hormone deficiency Type I	cDNA (growth hormone)
Haemophilia B	cDNA (Factor IX)
Lesch–Nyhan syndrome	cDNA (HPRT)
OTC deficiency	cDNA (ornithine transcarbanylase deficiency)
PKU	cDNA (phenylalanine hydroxylase)
Thalassaemia	cDNA (the β-globin cluster)

Restriction fragment length polymorphism in the human phenylalanine hydroxylase locus

As an example the gene coding for the enzyme phenylalanine hydroxylase (deficient in PKU) also consists of exons and introns, and the analytical procedure for prenatal diagnosis and carrier detection in PKU takes advantage of the benign nucleotide substitutions in the introns that can be detected by restriction endonucleases (Fig. 8.5). So, the patterns of DNA fragments obtained after digestion with restriction endonucleases are due to nucleotide substitutions in the non-coding sequences and are not responsible for the PKU phenotype.

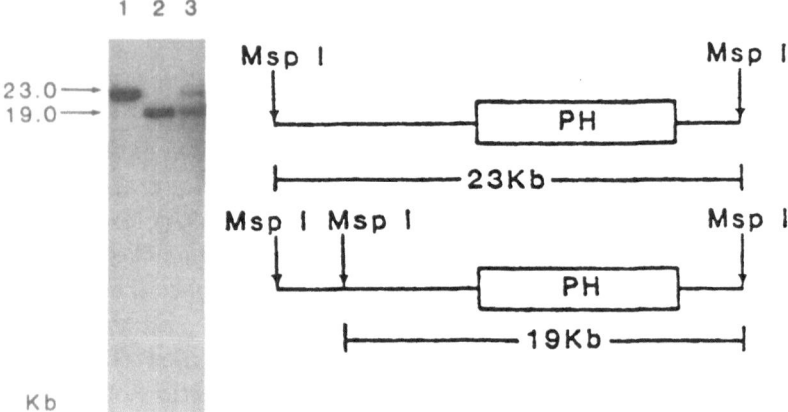

Figure 8.5 Profile of three selected individuals' DNA after digestion with the enzyme *MspI*. The explanation for this is schematically shown at the right-hand panel of the figure. Suppose that the phenylalanine hydroxylase gene in our genome detected by our cDNA probe is flanked by two *MspI* restriction sites that are 23 kb apart. During evolution there may have been a mutation contributing an additional *MspI* site at the 19 kb position. Individuals with two chromosomes of the 23 kb type will be homozygous for the 23 kb bands as shown in individual 1, and those with two chromosomes of the 19 kb type shown in lane 2 are homozygous for the 19 kb bands. If an individual has one each of the two chromosomes this individual will be a heterozygous for the 23 kb and 19 kb bands, respectively (lane 3)

Nevertheless, since the cDNA probes used in these analyses contain only the coding sequences of the gene itself, the detected polymorphisms exist either within, or immediately next to, the chromosomal gene[5]. Thus, the polymorphic patterns can be used for tracking of mutant genes in families by comparison of the parental and proband DNAs, and the analysis can be applied for prenatal diagnosis and carrier detection in these families (cf. Figs. 8.6 and 8.7).

In order to detect the existence of restriction fragment length polymorphism in the human phenylalanine hydroxylase locus, DNA was isolated from 20 random but otherwise normal individuals and analysed after digestion with a panel of restriction enzymes[5].

Figure 8.5 illustrates the restriction fragment length polymorphisms obtained with one restriction endonuclease, *Msp*I. But even additional restriction enzymes have revealed polymorphic patterns in the phenylalanine hydroxylase locus using a human phenylalanine hydroxylase cDNA probe[6].

Phenylalanine hydroxylase
gene region

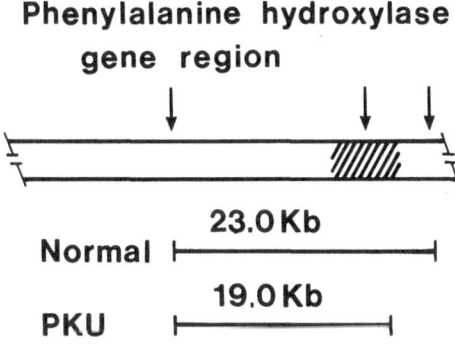

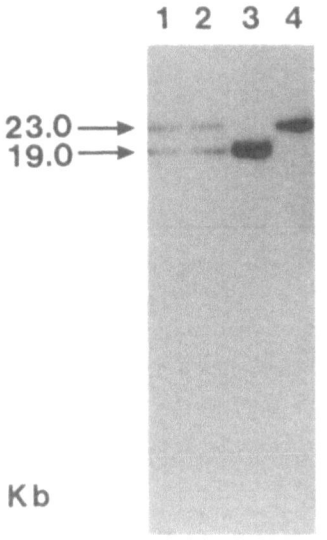

Figure 8.6 A Danish family's DNA after digestion with *Msp*I. It is obvious that both parents (lane 1 and 2) are heterozygous as both contain a band at 23 and 19 kb. If one looks at the DNA of the proband in lane 3 this individual is homozygous for the 19 kb band. Because PKU is an autosomal recessive disorder both parents may be obligate carriers and they must contain one copy of the mutant chromosome and one copy of the normal chromosome. By comparing the profiles of the two parents and the proband it can be concluded that the proband had inherited the two copies of the chromosomes of the 19 kb type and therefore these chromosomes are the mutant chromosomes of the family. By definition the 23 kb bands in the parents must carry the normal phenylalanine hydroxylase gene. These two genes have been transmitted to the unaffected sibling (lane 4), who is homozygous for the 23 kb band. This sibling is not only unaffected but free of the PKU trait

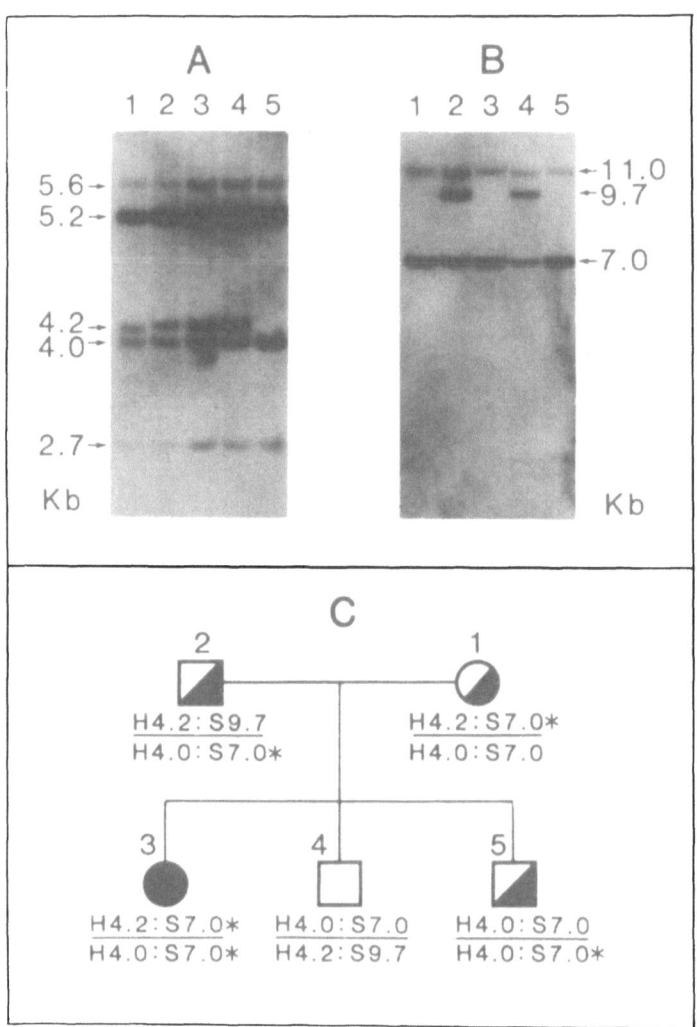

Figure 8.7   Haplotype analysis of the phenylalanine hydroxylase locus in a Danish PKU-family. 10 μg of DNA samples were digested with either *Hind*III (panel A) or *Sph*I (panel B) and applied to each lane in the gel as the following: lane 1, mother; lane 2, father; lane 3, proband; lane 4, an unaffected sibling; lane 5, a second unaffected sibling. Panel C: diagram showing the haplotypes of the phenylalanine hydroxylase gene for each family member and segregation of PKU-alleles (*) in this family[5]

KINDRED ANALYSIS OF CLASSICAL PKU FAMILIES

The existence of these allelic systems has permitted the analysis of classical PKU families by restriction fragment length polymorphisms. Leucocytes from Danish PKU families with one or two affected children and unaffected siblings were analysed. The low phenylalanine tolerance of the PKU children was ensured by frequent adjustments and recalculations. The combined phenotype of their parents based on phenylalanine loading tests was consistent with the prediction that their child suffered from classical PKU[7].

In the Danish families analysed so far with the partial-length human cDNA phenylalanine hydroxylase probe it has been possible to establish a linkage of the restriction fragment pattern with the mutant allele of the family.

From the example shown in Fig. 8.6 one can conclude that if this particular family have a pregnancy in the future it will be possible to offer a prenatal diagnosis by comparing the profiles that can be generated from the fetus DNA either by analysing the amniocytes or the chorionic biopsy villi trophoblasts. If the profiles are of type 4 in Fig. 8.6 the fetus will be free of the trait and if the profiles are one of type 1 or 2 in Fig. 8.6 the fetus will have inherited one of the mutant genes from the parents and one of the normal genes, and will therefore be a trait carrier.

In families with two affected children the segregation of the mutant allele and disease state has been concordant. Allelic segregation between the proband and unaffected siblings was discordant in all families. The powerful tool of haplotype analysis of the PKU-allele was documented[5, 8].

PRENATAL DIAGNOSIS OF PKU BY DNA ANALYSIS

It should be emphasized that the polymorphisms in the phenylalanine hydroxylase gene taken advantage of in this study are due to benign nucleotide substitutions in the gene and are not responsible for the PKU phenotype. Nevertheless, since the DNA probe used in these analyses is partially the one coding for phenylalanine hydroxylase itself, the detected polymorphism exists either within, or immediately next to, the chromosomal phenylalanine hydroxylase gene. Since the

DNA marker is so tightly linked to the phenylalanine hydroxylase gene, the probability of recombination between the polymorphic sites is insignificant. Thus, the polymorphic patterns can be used for tracking of mutant phenylalanine hydroxylase genes in PKU families by comparison of parental and proband DNAs, and prenatal diagnosis of PKU by polymorphism analysis is possible. So, the current technique for prenatal diagnosis rests on indirect evidence. However, we have recently performed the first prenatal diagnosis of PKU based on determination of the segregation of the mutant allele in the family. The diagnosis was confirmed when the mother gave birth to a PKU child. In another family the DNA analysis of amniotic fluid cells predicted a non-PKU child, which was also confirmed after delivery. These data demonstrate the specificity of this type of restriction endonuclease analysis (data to be published).

A phenylalanine hydroxylase full-length cDNA probe has revealed a high degree of restriction site polymorphism in the human genome

Recently a full-length DNA copy of the expressed part of the human gene for phenylalanine hydroxylase has been cloned. The nucleotide sequence of this cDNA gene has been determined. Furthermore, this cDNA clone contains the entire coding information for phenylalanine hydroxylase, since preliminary gene transfer studies demonstrate that it is capable of expressing authentic phenylalanine hydroxylase activity (data to be published). This finding allows cloning and sequence characterization of the normal and mutant phenylalanine hydroxylase genes in order to detect the structural mutations responsible for PKU. When the structural mutations in the phenylalanine hydroxylase gene responsible for PKU have been determined, specific oligonucleotides can be synthesized and used for prenatal diagnosis by direct analysis of the mutation sites in the gene isolated from amniotic fluid cells or chorionic villi trophoblasts, in the same way as specific oligonucleotides successfully have been used for detection of α_1-antitrypsin deficiency[9].

A panel of the commercially available restriction enzymes have revealed restriction site polymorphism in the human phenylalanine hydroxylase locus using the full-length (including all the nucleotide sequences of the exons) cDNA probe[10].

Most of these polymorphisms are spread in our population with a rather high frequency, e.g. the EcoRV polymorphism alone gives a heterozygosity of almost 50%. The theoretical haplotype hetero-zygosity, calculated using the frequencies of individual alleles, is well in excess of 95%.

Any given individual in the population will be either homozygous or heterozygous with respect to any of these alleles. The combination of the restriction patterns obtained after digestion of an individual's genomic DNA with each of the seven restriction enzymes makes a haplotype. Thus, a haplotype is the combination of the polymorphic restriction fragments or alleles obtained with different restriction enzymes.

By comparing the haplotype of the mutant phenylalanine hydroxy-lase gene of the PKU child with the haplotypes of the genomic DNA of the respective parents, who each have a normal and a mutant gene, it is possible for each parent to assign the haplotype associated with their normal gene and the haplotype associated with their mutant gene.

Using this strategy the haplotypes of 40 normal phenylalanine hydroxylase genes and 40 PKU genes have been determined. Out of a total of 1152 theoretical haplotypes, only 15 have actually been observed, suggesting that there may be a high degree of linkage dis-equilibrium between the polymorphic sites[10].

Of the 80 chromosomes analysed 64 were associated with the four haplotypes described in Table 8.2, and 16 chromosomes were asso-ciated with one of the 11 remaining haplotypes.

Table 8.2 Haplotypes associated with normal and mutant phenylalanine hydroxylase genes in Danish PKU heterozygotes*

Haplotype	Number of genes	
	Normal	PKU
1	15	8
2	1	10
3	3	13
4	10	4

* The data were compiled from 20 PKU families

Furthermore, in these preliminary investigations a majority of the PKU genes were associated with two of the four common haplotypes (haplotypes 2 and 3 in Table 8.2), both of which are different from the predominant haplotypes associated with the normal genes (haplotype 1 and 4 in Table 8.2). In order to demonstrate a significant association of specific haplotypes with specific phenylalanine hydroxylase genes, additional chromosomes will need to be analysed. However, the preliminary data shown in Table 8.2 suggest an association of distinct haplotypes with Danish PKU genes[10].

A high association of specific haplotypes with specific mutations in Mediterranean people with thalassaemia has been recently demonstrated[11]. The strong association between haplotype and mutation is somewhat surprising. It had previously been shown that since the same haplotypes associated with normal genes are found in different racial and ethnic groups, they must have originated before the divergence of the human races[11]. In contrast, as each ethnic group afflicted with β-thalassaemia has its own battery of mutations, these disease-producing mutations have occurred since the divergence of the races[11].

So, the association between haplotype and mutation may be due to a significant lapse of time between the occurrence of the first and any subsequent mutations on a particular chromosome background. On average, 86% of the mutations within a particular haplotype are identical, while 86% of the occurrence of a particular mutation are associated with a particular haplotype[11].

Based on these observations, and the assumption that a particular mutation is associated with a particular phenotype, it would be interesting to relate the various phenotypes of phenylalanine hydroxylase deficiency to the haplotypes associated with the mutant genes inherited from the parents.

DIRECT ANALYSIS OF GENETIC DISEASE USING SYNTHETIC OLIGONUCLEOTIDES

Recently the feasibility of using synthetic oligonucleotides to directly detect point mutations or nucleotide substitutions in the DNA has been explored in order to offer prenatal diagnosis for disorders where the base substitution responsible for the disease is known.

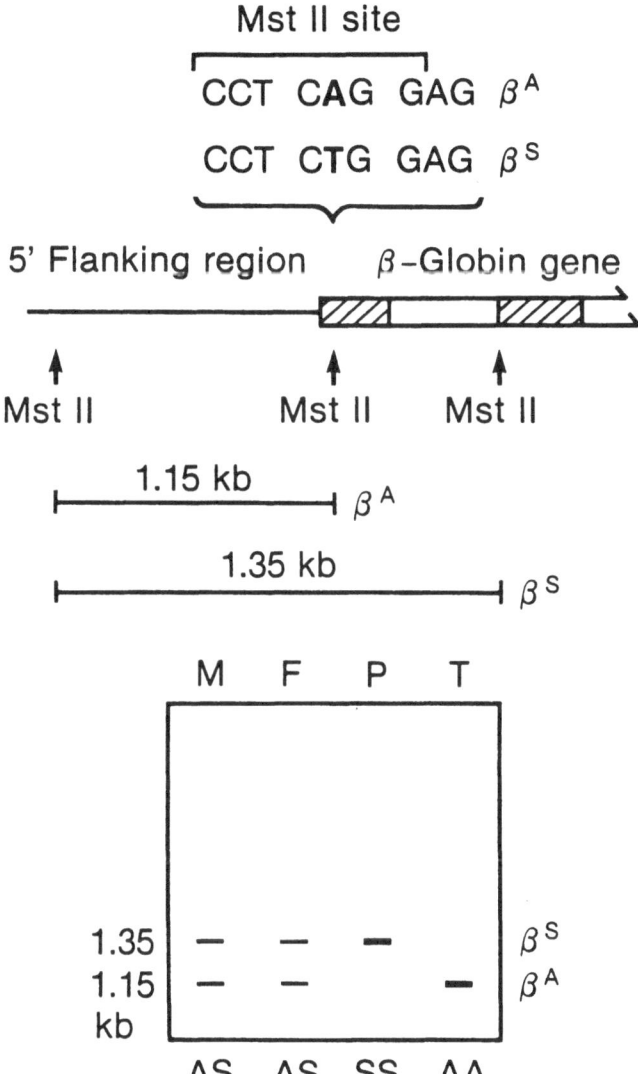

Figure 8.8 Diagnosis of sickle-cell anaemia by direct detection of the nucleotide substitution. The nucleotide sequence of the normal β^A-gene and the mutant sickle β^S-gene is shown at the top of the figure, including the *Mst*II cleavage site (CCTCAGG). The A → T substitutions in the β^S-gene alter the cleavage site for this restriction endonuclease. M, mother; F, father; P, proband; T, trophoblast DNA[12]

Table 8.3 Example of direct analysis of genetic disease using synthetic oligonucleotide to detect intragenic defects

Diseases	Probes
α_1-Antitrypsin deficiency	Synthetic oligonucleotide
Hereditary persistence of fetal haemoglobin	Synthetic oligonucleotide
HPRT deficiency (Lesch–Nyhan)	Synthetic oligonucleotide
Sickle-cell anaemia	Synthetic oligonucleotide
Thalassaemia	Synthetic oligonucleotide

Examples of genetic disease which can be analysed by direct analysis using gene probes to detect the intragenic defects are listed in Table 8.3.

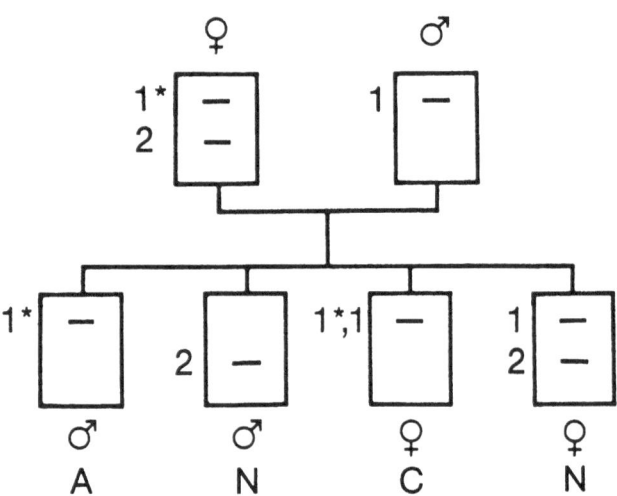

Figure 8.9 An example of linkage analysis of an X-linked disorder using a genomic DNA probe with a relatively short distance between the DNA sequence used as the probe and the mutant gene responsible for the disorder. The DNA restriction fragment 1* represents the restriction fragment with which the mutant gene on the X-chromosome segregates in the family. A: affected boy; N: unaffected boy; C: carrier daughter; N: normal daughter (cf. Ref. 13)

Indirect analysis of genetic disease using random genomic DNA probes to detect linked DNA polymorphism (Fig. 8.9)

Random genomic DNA probes containing both coding and non-coding (intervenient) nucleotide sequences close to the gene for Duchenne and Becker muscular dystrophies, as well as random DNA fragments close to the genes for Huntington's disease, X-linked retinitis pigmentosa, and fragile-X mental retardation syndrome, are being explored for linkage analysis.

Genetic disorders where random genomic DNA probes are used as DNA markers linked to the gene for the disorder have been reported (Table 8.4).

Table 8.4 Examples of indirect analysis of genetic disease using cloned DNA segments to detect linked DNA polymorphisms

Diseases	Probes
Fragile X-mental retardation syndrome	Factor IX[14]
Huntington's disease	G8 (chromosome 4)[15]
Muscular dystrophy	
Duchenne	RC8 + L1.28[13]
Becker	L1.28[16]

CONCLUSION

There are several limitations in these approaches to detection of the defect in certain single gene diseases[1]. Among these limitations are an error rate due to recombination during meiosis, non-random association between several polymorphic markers close to one another, the occurrence of similar genes in clusters (repeated copies), and the problem that it is not always possible to get complete digestion of the DNA with some restriction endonucleases. Complete digestion is mandatory for the diagnosis of genetic disorders by restriction endonuclease analysis of DNA.

An exponentially increasing number of cloned human DNA sequences are reported[17]. Thus, an increasing number of different genetic disorders can be diagnosed at the DNA level using restriction endonuclease fragment analysis. Some disorders can be diagnosed by detecting the defects (point mutations, deletions, additions and crossing-over products or hybrid genes) using appropriate restriction endonucleases and either synthetic oligonucleotides or cDNA probes, e.g. α_1-antitrypsin deficiency[9] or sickle-cell anaemia[12].

When the genetic defect at the DNA level is not yet detected DNA polymorphisms can be used to differentiate between the chromosome carrying a normal gene and the chromosome carrying the mutant gene. When linkage between the mutant gene and the DNA fragments obtained has been established in a family, carrier detection and pre-natal diagnosis can be offered using a cDNA sequence as the probe and appropriate restriction endonucleases to obtain informative restriction fragment polymorphisms.

The possibility for the diagnosis of the genetic disorders mentioned above implies that probes specific for those genes which are defective are available (cDNA gene probes, synthetic oligonucleotides). For genetic diseases in which the gene is not known, such as Duchenne muscular dystrophy, Huntington's disease or cystic fibrosis, it may be possible to correlate the presence or absence of the putative abnormal gene with a restriction endonuclease polymorphism and therefore be able to mark the abnormal gene with a specific pattern of polymorphism[13-16]. The progress that has been made with the detection of polymorphisms very closely linked to the putative abnormal genes suggests that the sequences that contain the abnormal genes might be isolated in the near future. In that case specific probes will become available and furthermore the basic defects identified. Recombinant DNA technology is already having great impact in the study of the basic defect causing several types of disorders in haematology, endocrinology, hereditary connective tissue diseases, immunology, infectious disease, and oncology, and will soon play an important role in other common disorders such as hypertension and the genetic basis of atherosclerosis.

ACKNOWLEDGEMENT

The Danish Medical Research Council, the Danish Health Insurance Foundation, the Danish Mental Retardation Service, and the P. Carl Pedersen's Fund have supported the author's contributions to this review.

REFERENCES

1. Antonarakis, S. E., Phillips, J. A. and Kazazian, H. H. (1982). Genetic diseases: diagnosis by restriction endonuclease analysis. *J. Pediatr.*, **100**, 845–56
2. Editorial (1984). Molecular genetics for the clinician. *Lancet*, **1**, 257–9
3. Messer, A. and Porter, I. H. (eds.) (1983). *Recombinant DNA and Medical Genetics*. (New York, London: Academic Press)
4. Nathans, D. and Smith, H. O. (1975). Restriction endonucleases in the analysis and restructuring of DNA molecules. *Ann. Rev. Biochem.*, **44**, 273–82
5. Woo, S. L. C., Lidsky, A. S., Güttler, F., Chandra, T. and Robson, K. J. H. (1983). Cloned human phenylalanine hydroxylase gene allows prenatal diagnosis and carrier detection of classical phenylketonuria. *Nature*, **306**, 151–5
6. Woo, S. L. C., Güttler, F., Ledley, F. D., Lidsky, A. S., DiLella, A. G., Kwork, S. C. M. and Robson, K. J. H. (1985). The human phenylalanine hydroxylase gene. I. In Berg, K. (ed.) *Medical Genetics: Past, Present, Future*. (New York: Allan R. Liss) (In press)
7. Güttler, F. (1980). Hyperphenylalaninemia: diagnosis and classification of the various types of phenylalanine hydroxylase deficiency in childhood. *Acta Paediatr. Scand.*, Suppl. **280**, 1–80
8. Woo, S. L. C., Lidsky, A. S., Güttler, F., Thirumalachary, C. and Robson, K. J. H. (1984). Prenatal diagnosis of classical phenylketonuria by gene mapping. *J. Am. Med. Assoc.*, **251**, 1998–2002
9. Kidd, V. J., Golbus, M. S., Wallace, R. B., Itakura, K. and Woo, S. L. C. (1984). α_1-Antitrypsin deficiency detection by direct analysis of the mutation in the gene. *N. Engl. J. Med.*, **300**, 639–42
10. Güttler, F., Woo, S. L. C. and Lidsky, A. (1985). Molecular genetics of PKU: prenatal diagnosis and carrier detection by gene analysis. I. In Bickel, H. (ed.) *Recent Progress in the Understanding, Recognition and Management of Inherited Diseases of Amino Acid Metabolism*. (Stuttgart and New York: Thieme) (In press)
11. Kazazian, Jr., H. H., Orkin, S. H., Markham, A. F., Chapman, C. R., Youssoufian, H. and Waber, P. G. (1984). Quantification of the close association between DNA haplotypes and specific β-thalassaemia mutations in Mediterraneans. *Nature*, **310**, 152–4
12. Orkin, S. H., Little, P. F. R., Kazazian, Jr., H. H. and Boehm, C. D. (1982). Improved detection of the sickle mutation by DNA analysis. Application to prenatal diagnosis. *N. Engl. J. Med.*, **307**, 32–6
13. Pembrey, M. E., Davies, K. E., Winter, R. M., Elles, R. G., Williamson, R., Fazzone, T. A. and Walker, C. (1984). Clinical use of DNA markers linked to the gene for Duchenne muscular dystrophy. *Arch. Dis. Child.*, **59**, 208–16

14. Camerino, G., Mattei, M. G., Mattei, J. F., Jaye, M. and Mandel, J. L. (1983). Close linkage of fragile X-mental retardation syndrome to haemophilia B and transmission through a normal male. *Nature*, **306**, 701–4

15. Gusella, J. F., Wexler, N. S., Conneally, P. M. *et al.* (1983). A polymorphic DNA marker genetically linked to Huntington's disease. *Nature*, **306**, 234–8

16. Kingston, H. M., Thomas, N. S. T., Pearson, P. L., Sarfarazi, M. and Harper, P. S. (1983). Genetic linkage between Becker muscular dystrophy and a polymorphic DNA sequence on the short arm of the X-chromosome. *J. Med. Genet.*, **20**, 255–8

17. Schmidtke, J. and Cooper, D. N. (1984). A list of cloned human DNA sequences. *Hum. Genet.*, **67**, 111–14

9
Acid phosphatase and heterologous gene expression in yeast

H. RUDOLPH and A. HENNEN

Saccharomyces cerevisiae (yeast) is one of the best understood eukaryotic organisms. The fact that this unicellular micro-organism has a short generation time and is easy to grow under defined culture conditions has made it a favoured object for biochemical and genetic studies for several decades. More recently the newly elaborated yeast gene cloning techniques have made it possible to extend their analysis to the molecular level.

We chose the acid phosphatase gene family in order to study gene expression in yeast. The basic characterization of this system is in progress and will provide us with necessary information about the genes and the signals which regulate their expression. Two of the structural genes, the regulated *PHO5* gene and the constitutively expressed *PHO3* gene, have been isolated and sequenced.

Using the DNA sequence data we have built a yeast expression vector and we have achieved expression of several foreign genes in yeast under the control of the *PHO5* promoter. Three different α-interferon genes (types D, B, F) have been fused in the middle of their respective N-terminal signal sequences with the beginning of the *PHO5* signal sequence and the adjacent *PHO5* promoter. More than 80% of the interferon protein shows the molecular weight of mature interferon. The exact processing site is currently being analysed. Several modifications in the presumed mRNA termination area have increased the levels of D-type interferon expression above 1% of the total soluble protein in a yeast cell extract. In addition, we have obtained high levels of expression for hepatitis surface antigen. Yeast seems to be a particularly good host for the expression of this protein since it is, up to now, the only micro-organism able to assemble the individual proteins into a spherical particle with immunogenic properties similar to the native virus.

Part 3
MONOCLONAL ANTIBODIES: ADVANTAGES AND DISADVANTAGES

10
Monoclonal antibodies as research tools

A. E. BUSSARD

The establishment of permanent immunoclones in 1975 marks one of the major landmarks in the history of immunology; the other one, contemporary to it, being the development of molecular immunology and the concept of minigenes.

The significance of the monoclonal antibodies (MA) methodology as a research tool can be seen in two directions: internal and external to immunology.

The internal direction concerns the use of this methodology to analyse the immune response. For the first time in history we are in the position to dissect the immune repertoire, and we are already reassessing our views about the size of this repertoire. This size is probably three orders of magnitude larger than what was accepted even 10 years ago. Consequently MA provide tools of an exquisite specificity for the detection of the innumerable epitopes available.

In fact the similarity between the size of the repertoire of epitopes and the size of the immune repertoire reflects the adaptation of the higher vertebrate's immune system to the ever-increasing diversity of the antigens they encounter.

A first practical conclusion is that, if the diversity of antibodies is of the order of 10^8, and if the immunologists manufacture 10^4 new MA every year (this is a reasonable estimate) it will require 10^4 years before we can cover the Universe of antibodies! The consequence is that the storing of the information regarding the MA available can only be dealt with by computerized systems. This is why we are in the process of establishing a computerized Hybridoma Data Bank (HDB).

Another aspect of the internal use of MA in immunology concerns their applications to the study of antibody biosynthesis at the molecular and cellular level: molecular mechanisms involved in the genes assortment from nuclear DNA to the final cytoplasmic RNA, analysis of the mRNA from hybridomas, chains assembly, mechanisms of antibody secretion, etc.; all problems of molecular immunology which were, till now, studied on myeloma cells, can be studied on cells producing antibodies of a chosen specificity. MA can also be used, for external reasons, as immunological tools for the study of a large number of problems: detection of epitopes (diagnostic probes in medicine, parasitology, agriculture, biochemistry, organic chemistry), analysis of the structure of molecules (enzymes, hormones . . .), etc., but also for preparative goals (purification of virus, interferon, organic compounds, etc.).

MA are also used for both internal and external reasons: the study of the immunoglobulin itself: general structure, allotypes, idiotopes, isotopes and paratopes.

MA are exquisitely specific reagents and like many other modern biotechnological tools they represent a considerable advance but they also have some drawbacks. These drawbacks are minor as long as the users of these reagents are conscious of some of their limitations, and know the basic principles involved in their use.

It is therefore of importance to consider some characteristics of the MA which underline their limits of application and also to mention some of the efforts made to establish a catalogue of the already enormous mass of these reagents.

PURITY OF MONOCLONAL ANTIBODIES

MA are generally produced either as tissue culture supernatants or as ascitic fluid from mice bearing hybridomas. In the first case the crude tissue culture supernatant contains from 10 to 50 μg of specific antibody with the order of 3–5 mg of proteins from fetal calf serum, or horse serum if the sera were used at 10% final concentration. It means that the specific antibody represents from 0.3 to 1.7% of the total protein content. The culture fluid can be used as such or can be purified either as Ig preparation (salt precipitation of protein A adsorption, if the subclass of the MA is convenient) or as specific antibody by immunochromatography.

In some cases for instance, tissue culture can be performed in the absence of protein, for some rat–rat hybridomas. The search for a universal protein-free tissue culture medium, applicable to all kinds of hybridomas, is going on all over the world but as far as is known has not yet succeeded.

The other way to obtain MA results is from the transplantation of hybridoma cells in the peritoneal cavity of histocompatible mice. With this technique a much higher yield of specific MA can be attained: of the order of 10–20 mg of MA per ml of serum (a thousand times the yield of tissue culture). Nevertheless one must keep in mind that a mouse is not a simple incubator; it is a living body, producing and exporting in the peritoneal fluid its own proteins and immunoglobulins. Consequently the MA are diluted by proteins and immunoglobulins from the mouse bearing the hybridomas. Indeed, with the high potential of multiplication and secretion of the hybridomas, MA may represent 50–70 % of the immunoglobulins of the ascitic fluid. A further purification by immunochromatography could get rid of the extraneous Ig. Unfortunately, there is one case where it is impossible to purify the MA by specific means: this is when the ascitic fluid contains natural antibodies produced by the mouse directed against the same antigens as the one recognized by the MA. This possibility is not a theoretical one, but has been found in the case of anti-peroxidase antibodies which are present in the ascitic fluid from normal mice. There is no way to purify, with immunoadsorption columns, these ascitic fluids, since both MA from the hybridomas and the natural polyclonal antibodies from the mouse will be retained by the column. In some very limited cases, separation of the MA from the polyclonal antibodies can be achieved if these two families of Ig are from different subclasses but this cannot be a general procedure.

In summary, one or the other procedure for obtaining MA should be chosen in reference to the problem to be solved and by taking due consideration of the possible contamination of MA in ascitic fluid by natural antibodies.

What is essential, however, is that the users must be aware of the nature of the reagent they are employing, its source (tissue culture fluid, ascitic fluid, etc.), its concentration, the species it comes from and its isotype.

SPECIFICITY OF MONOCLONAL ANTIBODIES

It is commonly thought by non-immunologists that, since MA have an exquisite specificity, they cannot be cross-reactive. This is based on confusion regarding the concept of cross-reaction.

Cross-reaction relates to the possibility for a paratope (antibody combining site) to react not only with the epitope (antigenic site) against which it has been raised (tri-nitro-phenol (TNP) for example) but also against epitopes which are structurally related to it di-nitro-phenol (DNP) in the former example). Naturally, MA, though they are a homogeneous family of molecules, can cross-react with different epitopes, as predicted. The useful characteristic of an hybridization is that it can give rise to some MA which, for a given epitope, may not cross-react with another one structurally related. This should be demonstrated for each MA examined.

Unfortunately cross-reactivity is a term loosely used to characterize the polyspecificity of polyclonal sera, but this has nothing to do with the true cross-reactivity, as defined previously. This polyspecificity reveals the polyclonality of a serum raised against a given antigen. This serum behaves like a mixture of MA, the different families of antibodies reacting with different epitopes of the immunogen.

Nevertheless it is to be expected that, in terms of true cross-reactivity, MA can react with two different molecules, if they have some structural similarities.

SURVEY OF THE EXISTING MONOCLONAL ANTIBODIES

The number of possible applications of MA is already enormous. Such a wide field of applications naturally has attracted considerable interest among potential users. Consequently, the production of IC and MA have risen rapidly in the past 5 years so that the number of reagents available today is very large; around 5×10^4 – but is very difficult to estimate. The annual production of new MA must be approaching 10^4!

It is thus impossible for a potential user (whether in the academic field or industry) to discover if a given MA has already been produced, by whom and where it can be obtained. Unavoidable duplication of effort results in serious loss of money and time since the cost of establishing a given Immunoclone (IC) has been estimated to be of the order of $25,000 and 6 months duration. It seems obvious that some kind of a list of extant MA and IC should be established and made available to the scientific community. This catalogue should meet the following minimum requirements:

1. It should be international in scope for entries and for distribution of information.
2. It should be computerized.
3. It should be easily accessible to everybody.
4. Its cost should be cheap.

The first point is related to the fact that the seekers of MA or IC are unconcerned by the nationality of the producer. Building data banks at the national, then regional, and finally international levels, would be a waste of time, engender duplication of information and would be a costly procedure. It is much wiser to establish a central data bank immediately at an international level, for the collection and storage of data.

In contrast to the collection and storage of data, the distribution (output) of information in answer to queries may use a decentralized structure of 'satellites' or 'nodes' at a regional or national level.

The second requirement, that it be computerized, seems to be an obvious consequence of the anticipated number of MA and IC, the number of categories of information on each, and the need for rapid, easy retrieval of various combinations of data. Questions might be on the nature of fusion partners, availability of products, specificity, affinity, class of the Ig, etc. Different queries will be satisfied by the use of various combinations of search parameters. Such a flexible search system can be achieved realistically only by computerization of the data, using a specialized program established by experts.

The third requirement will be met through the use of the computer from the central bank or from geographically distributed centres. The creation of such a bank has been undertaken jointly by the Committee on Data for Science and Technology (CODATA) and the International Union of Immunological Societies (IUIS), both members of the International Council of Scientific Unions. The central office of the data bank (HDB) is:

CODATA/IUIS Hybridoma Data Bank, Ms. Lois Blaine, 12301 Parklawn Drive, Rockville, Maryland 20852, USA.

The policies, planning, and monitoring of performance of the HDB are the responsibilities of a formally constituted Task Group of CODATA. This Task Group comprises the following members: Prof. A. Bussard, Chairman (France); Dr R. Accolla (Switzerland);

Dr G. Hammerling (FRG); Dr V. Houba (WHO); Dr B. Janicki (USA); Dr M. Krichevsky, Secretary (USA); Dr E. S. Lennox (UK); Dr J. Natvig (Norway); and Dr T. Tada (Japan).

The following organizations are already contributing funds to the bank: Institute for Physical and Chemical Research (Japan); United States National Institutes of Health (NIAID, NIDR, NIGMS, NCI, NIGMS, DRR), Food and Drug Administration (USA); American Type Culture Collection (USA); Medical Research Council (UK); Mission Interministérielle de l'Information Scientifique et Technique (France); Fonds National Suisse; World Health Organization; Committee on Data for Science and Technology and the International Union of Immunological Societies.

One main element in the success of such a data bank is the structure of the system used for information storage. The system chosen for the HDB is the NIDR/FDA Microbial Information System (MICRO-IS). The MICRO-IS is designed to manage large volumes of individual microbial strain information. Adaptation of the system to MA and IC information required only minor programming changes.

Information is submitted by IC and MA producers on a specialized data reporting form (DRF). The main characteristics of this DRF are that it is easily understood, flexible in format, and open-ended, in order to be able to cope with individual laboratory situations and the unpredictable directions of progress of the technology in the field of cellular biology.

Another element contributing to the success of the bank is the amount of data collected relative to the amount of the total existing data. To maximize this ratio the HDB will use some original means of collecting the data, such as seeking the collaboration of editors of scientific journals as contacts for data contribution from authors of relevant papers.

The progress of the bank is followed regularly by the Task Group, and its value will be assessed after 3 years of existence to decide upon its future.

The field of IC is of considerable importance both for basic and for applied research. Its economical bearings are very large (the present budget of the MA industry is in the order of 10^8) and the future is very promising. We hope that the establishment of this bank will further help development in this field.

11
Monoclonal antibodies: advantages and disadvantages in production of test systems

W. H. W. ALBERT

INTRODUCTION

Conventionally prepared antibodies have been used for many years as research tools and for diagnostic and therapeutic purposes. They have been useful reagents in many respects, although their application has sometimes been limited by their inherent biochemical properties. If an animal is immunized with an immunogenic substance, a whole range of predetermined cell clones belonging to the class of B-lympho-cytes is activated, induced to proliferate, and triggered to synthesize antibodies.

There are usually several molecular structures – so-called epitopes – on an antigenic entity. Each of them is able to elicit an immune response. A great variety of different antibody molecules are thus induced. Even against one epitope antibodies with different affinities and binding characteristics are formed. This can in many instances cause problems if very high specificity, or if consistent quality of the antibody reagent, are desired. The reproducibility of antiserum quality is additionally hampered by the fact that each animal, even when derived from an inbred strain, shows a different pattern of antibody response. This response varies not only from animal to animal but also changes during the life span of an individual.

Therefore, when Köhler and Milstein[1] succeeded in producing monoclonal antibodies (MA) with predetermined specificity, a great step towards the perfection of immune reagents was achieved. This invention paved the way to continuous, virtually limitless, production of antibodies with selected and well-characterized specificities. Antibodies can now be obtained which will react in a reproducible fashion with any known antigen or hapten.

The problems related to the use of MA in test development will now be reviewed.

ANTIBODY AFFINITY

Because of the need to determine many disease markers or drugs at a low concentration in body fluids or tissue specimens, and because of the trend towards shortening the time needed to perform clinical assays, antibodies with high affinity for a given ligand are needed. This often requires a long search for a suitable clone producing antibodies with the desired affinity and specificity. The animal most commonly used for immunization and cell hybridization is the inbred Balb/c mouse, whose immune response to certain antigens is sometimes inferior to other mouse strains or other species. Thus sometimes – but fortunately rarely – an insufficient immune response against a particular immunogen is seen. In this case choosing a different mouse strain or a different species – for instance the rat – for immunization might help. Also making cross-species hybridomas can be advantageous. However there is the tendency to eliminate the genes coding for the antibody.

An often underestimated aspect in the development of monoclonal antibodies with high affinity is the immunization protocol: the addition and choice of adjuvants, the application site, the antigen dose, the frequency of application and the duration of immunization can be of prime importance. In our experience it has been advantageous to immunize for a long period. The best yield of high affinity antibodies was obtained after at least 4 months immunization.

Here, the phenomenon of affinity maturation[2-4] should be mentioned. This theory describes a selection process for high affinity antibody-producing clones through antigenic stimulation over a long period. Thereby clones which bind to the antigen with higher affinity are preferably stimulated by antigens to proliferate, leaving other clones with lower affinity without antigenic challenge. Combined with somatic mutation this effect will lead to a selection in favour of clones producing high-affinity antibodies. An observation we have made is that high affinity alone is not always a guarantee for a good performance in a given test system.

The rate of formation of a ligand–antibody complex is dependent on the concentration of the reaction partners, ligand and antibody, and two constants described as association rate and dissociation rate constant as defined by the mass action law. We can discriminate between high-affinity and low-affinity systems: in the high-affinity system certain features can be observed. On the one hand, slow association and slow dissociation rates can lead to high affinity. On the other hand, very fast association and fast dissociation rates can do the same. This means that the determination of the affinity constant, for instance by Scatchard plot analysis, might not tell you how the antibody behaves in a situation where the dissociation rate becomes important for the test design. This I will try to show later on.

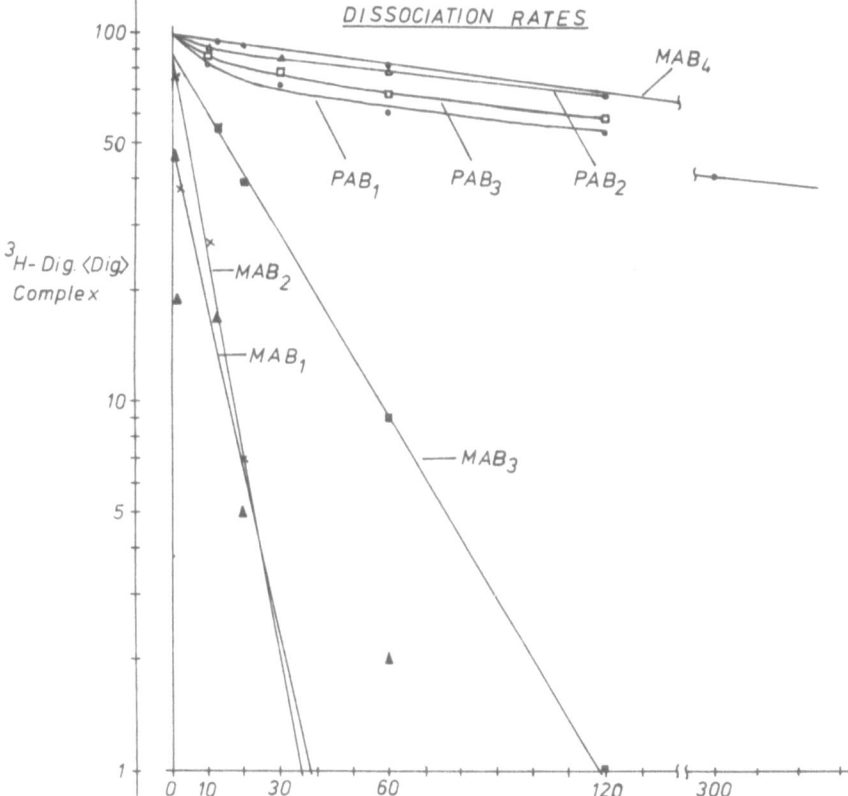

Figure 11.1 Dissociation rates of several monoclonal antibodies (MA) and polyclonal antibodies (PA) having a similar overall high affinity to the digoxin

Comparison of the dissociation rates of several monoclonal and polyclonal antibodies (PA) having a similar overall high affinity towards the drug digoxin (Fig. 11.1) showed that most of the monoclonal antibodies tested have a rather fast dissociation rate with a half-time under 30 min, whereas the three polyclonal antibodies have a very slow dissociation rate with a half-time over several hours. Only one monoclonal antibody performs similarly to the polyclonal antibodies. This finding has practical consequences in that MA are often inferior to PA in the so called 1-site radio- or enzyme-immunometric assay.

In this type of assay a surplus of insolubilized ligand is usually employed to remove labelled antibodies not saturated by the soluble ligand. If the dissociation rate is fast, the surplus of insoluble ligand can cause a shift in the equilibrium. The dissociated antibody molecules then preferably bind to the insolubilized ligand. This will lower the test performance. It is thus necessary and worthwhile to carefully study the kinetics of the antibody binding before selecting a MA for a particular test system.

ANTIBODY AVIDITIES

If at least two antibodies, preferably preselected MA, are able to bind to two independent epitopes of an antigen, a cyclic complex can be formed. This has proven to be the most stable configuration of an antigen–antibody complex. If dissociation takes place on one or even two binding sites, the complex will not dissolve entirely and re-association can take place. This increase in avidity up to 100-fold and more can only happen if intact antibodies or at least (Fab)$_2$ fragments with two binding sites are used[5,6].

Cross-reactivity has become much more transparent since we were able to use monoclonal antibodies.

CROSS-REACTIVITY

An hypothesis by N. Jerne states that there are far more antibody specifications than antibody-producing clones *and* antibodies. The logical consequence had to be that one antibody can have more than

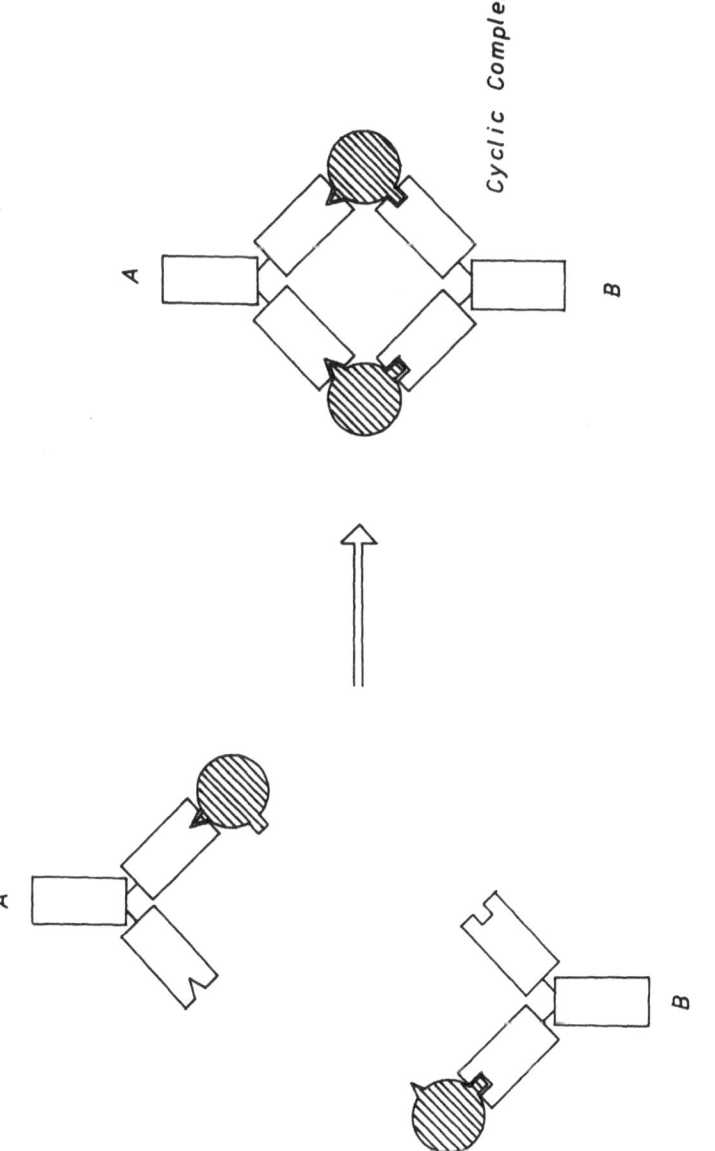

Figure 11.2 Method of increasing antibody avidity[6]

one binding region[7-10]. This means that one can still be surprised by seemingly paradoxical results related to cross-reactivity even when using monoclonal antibodies.

When discussing cross-reactivity I would like to use the terms as suggested by Berzofsky and Schechter[11], namely 'true' cross-reactivity and 'shared' cross-reactivity. 'True' cross-reactivity means that ligand and cross-reacting ligand are bound by the same antibody binding site, but with different affinities. This situation is typical for MA. 'Shared' cross-reactivity is observed with PA. They are heterogeneous with respect to epitopes they recognize but also with respect to affinities within a subpopulation of antibodies reacting with each single epitope.

If antiserum or antibody is absorbed by a ligand, unreacted antibody will diminish with increasing concentration of the ligand. If the affinity to a 'truly' cross-reacting ligand is lower, more ligand is needed to absorb the unreacted antibody. However, when only 'shared' cross-reactivity of the ligand towards polyclonal antibodies is present, only the antibody fraction reacting with this 'shared' epitope can be absorbed out. There remains an antibody activity which cannot be absorbed by the cross-reacting ligand.

Association and dissociation rates are important for test design as mentioned before. Let us consider the situation illustrated in Figs. 11.3 and 11.4. A given amount of antibody A $(2.5 \times 10^{-10}\,mol/l)$ is reacting with the corresponding ligand B $(5 \times 10^{-10}\,mol/l)$ to form a ligand–antibody complex D. The association constant is 10^7, the dissociation constant 10^{-4}. We can now simulate the reaction kinetics, that means the time-dependent formation of the ligand–antibody complex D, by a computer program.

Imagine now that a cross-reactive substance is present in a 10-fold higher concentration; but association and dissociation constants are slightly different. One can see that the formation of the product E, that is of the complex of antibody and cross-reacting ligand, is very prominent during the first 5 min. The 'first come, first served' effect shows clearly. Only after 20 min can we determine ligand B without gross interference through ligand C. If we change nothing but the association constant between antibody and cross-reacting ligand C by a factor of 10 a dramatic change in the reaction pattern occurs: the test becomes totally unspecific even at equilibrium. This shows again that the study of antibody kinetics is of great importance in test design, especially when MA are employed.

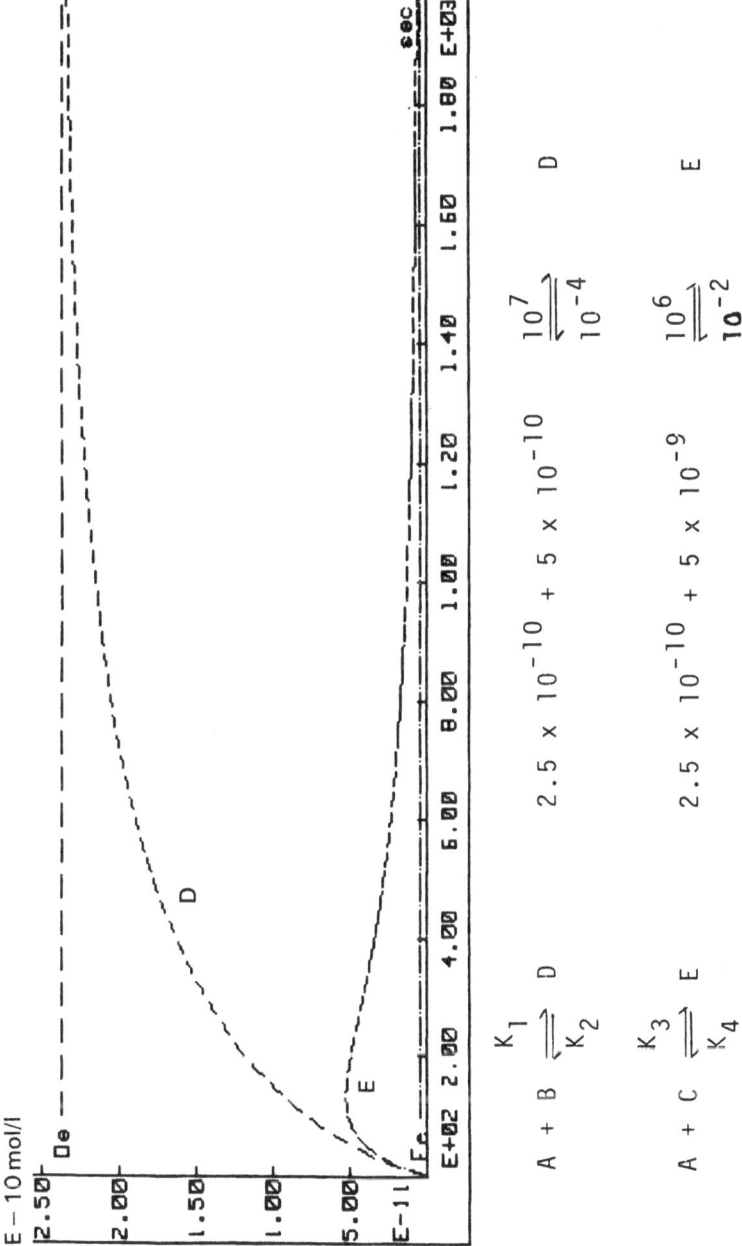

Figure 11.3 Time-dependent formation of the ligand–antibody complex D and the cross-reacting ligand–antibody complex E

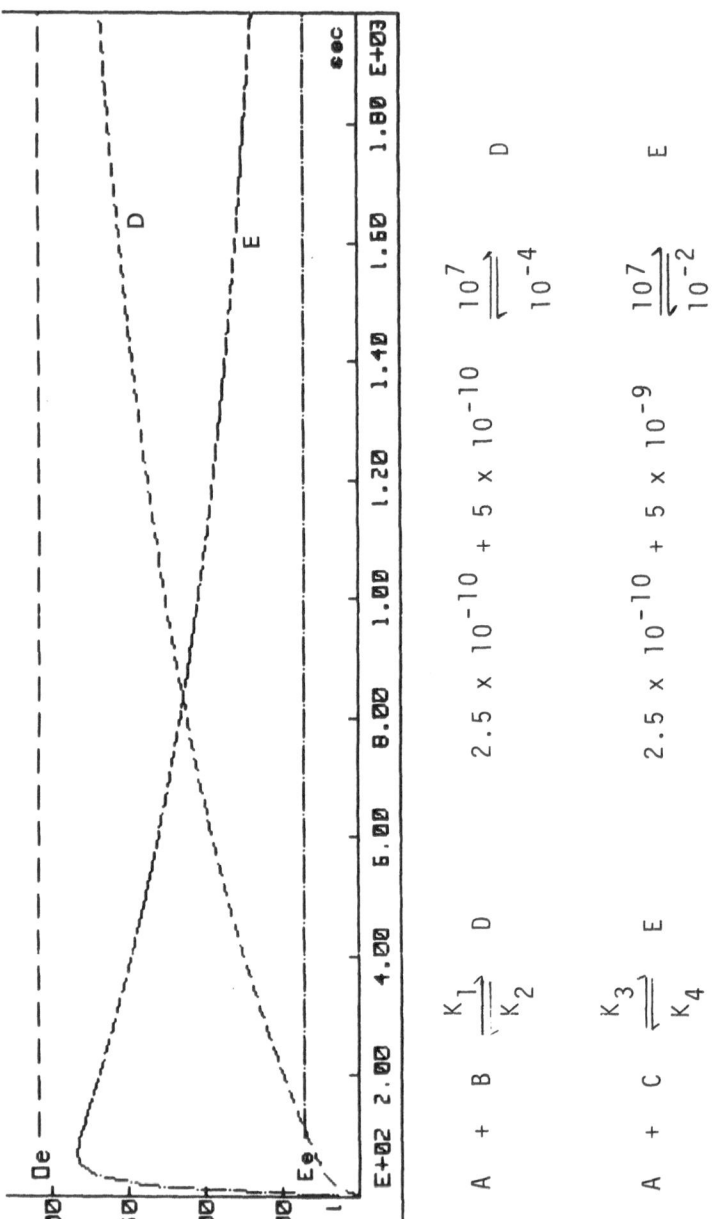

Figure 11.4   Time-dependent formation of the ligand–antibody complex D and the cross-reacting ligand–antibody complex E

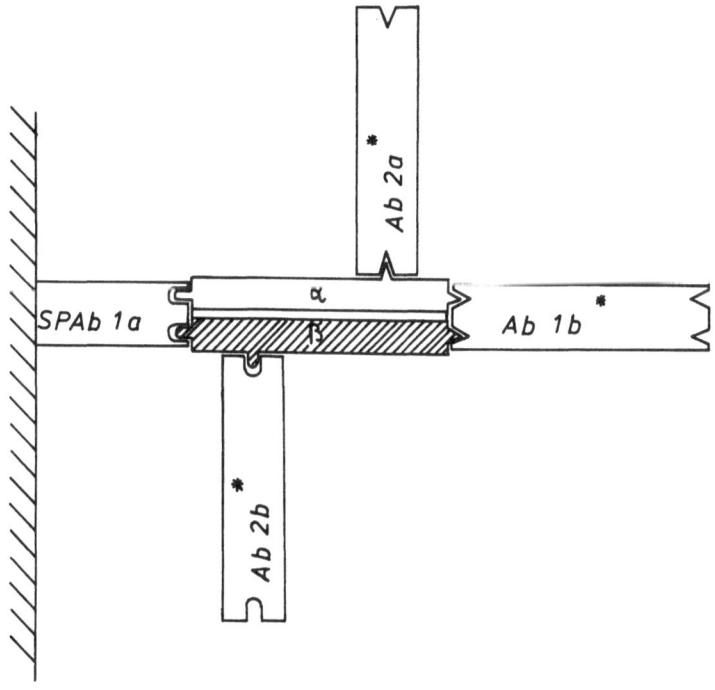

Figure 11.5 Cross-reactivity: specific test for peptide hormone MA. Antibodies *1a* and *1b* are conformation-specific; single α- or β-chains are not recognized. *Ab* = antibody; *SPAB* = solid phase antibody; *Ab** = labelled antibody

DEVELOPMENT OF MA FOR PEPTIDE HORMONES

Many of these hormones consist of a hormone-specific β-chain and a common α-chain. Only α- and β-chain combined are biologically active; but only the β-chain has peptide sequences characteristic for a particular hormone. We tried, for instance, to select a monoclonal antibody specific for the biologically active TSH molecule and succeeded. We obtained similar results with HCG. That means that there are structural epitopes only present in native hormones. This is very important if the amount of biologically active hormone has to be determined.

A specific test for one of those hormones can be designed as shown in Fig. 11.5. Monoclonal antibody specific for the native, intact antigen is bound to a solid phase; labelled monoclonal or polyclonal antibody is used as marker. The amount of antigen bound to the solid phase antibody is directly related to the signal generated by the second labelled antibodies. This test design is frequently referred to as sandwich type assay. The specificity achieved by this test design in the case of a TSH-test was such that no cross-reactivity with any hormone structurally related to TSH could be observed.

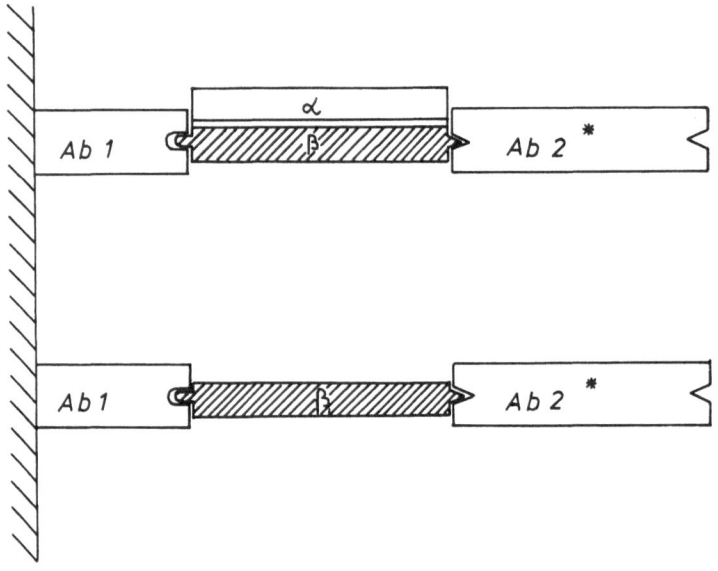

Figure 11.6   Cross-reactivity: specific test for β-chain MA. Antibodies *1* and *2** are β-chain specific; single α-chains are not recognized

A different situation exists when the β-chain, for instance for HCG, should be determined as a tumour associated marker (Fig. 11.6). Only free β-chain, as found with certain tumours, *together* with the native hormone, can be determined. It becomes apparent that a careful selection of antibodies for a particular purpose is of utmost importance. In my opinion an HCG-test, being β-chain specific, is of limited value for pregnancy testing but certainly useful for tumour monitoring.

Monoclonal antibodies have unique biochemical and physical properties. The influence of pH, ionic strength and other environmental factors may be of much greater importance to their physical behaviour than to PA, where most of the time some antibody subpopulation will still function orderly.

CHANGES IN EPITOPES ON ANTIGEN

Not only antibodies are susceptible to environmental changes; epitopes on antigens can also be modulated or even disappear. The modulation or disappearance of epitopes can lead to an underestimation of antigen concentration (Fig. 11.7). We believed that α-fetoprotein is a reasonably stable antigen. But when we tested a combination of two monoclonal antibodies in a sandwich-type assay we had to accept the fact that one epitope was labile after prolonged storage. Other examples are MA against human immunoglobulins, which performed well in radio- or enzyme-immunoassays but gave inferior results in immunohistochemistry, probably due to denaturing of epitopes by the fixation procedure[12].

PROTEOLYSIS

Proteolysis may also play a role in the underestimation of proteins with MA as compared to PA (Fig. 11.8). These findings also have implications for the characterization of reference material and of calibrators used to standardize test reagents. Careful studies of the stabilities of antigens, and even of epitopes reacting with monoclonal antibodies, have to be made. Appropriate environmental or matrix conditions have to be defined for the optimal performance of ligand–antibody reactions. For peptide hormones, for example, an exact quantitation of native hormone and isolated α- and β-chain in the reference material should be performed.

For the development of test reagents the screening system for MA should be designed in such a way that it is compatible with the end-use; i.e. one should know exactly what one wants to assay and how one wants to determine the antigens or haptens and then screen accordingly.

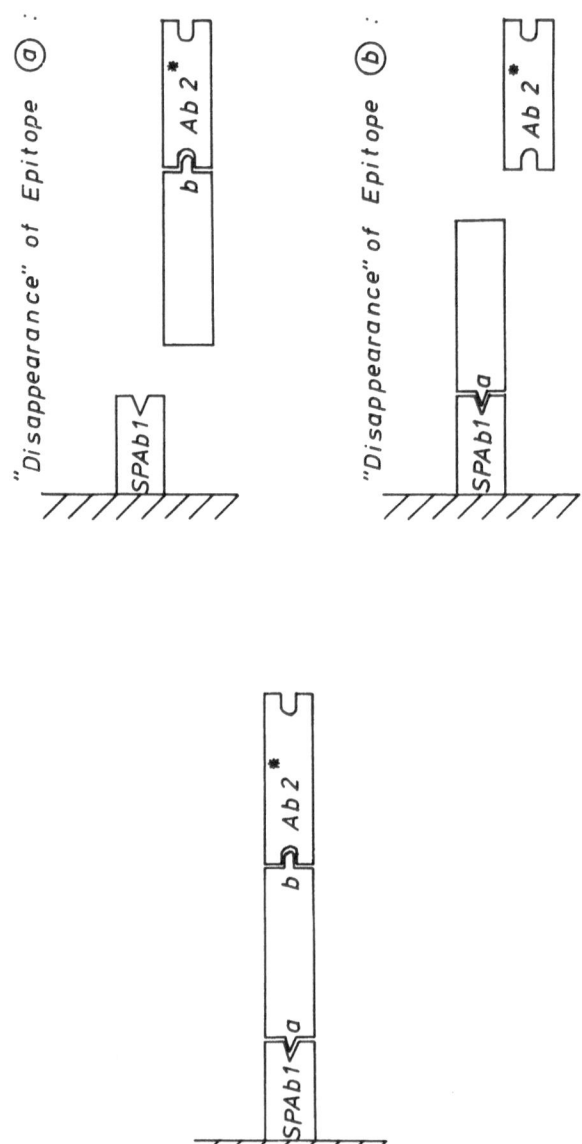

Figure 11.7 Structural epitopes: influence of pH, ionic strength or others

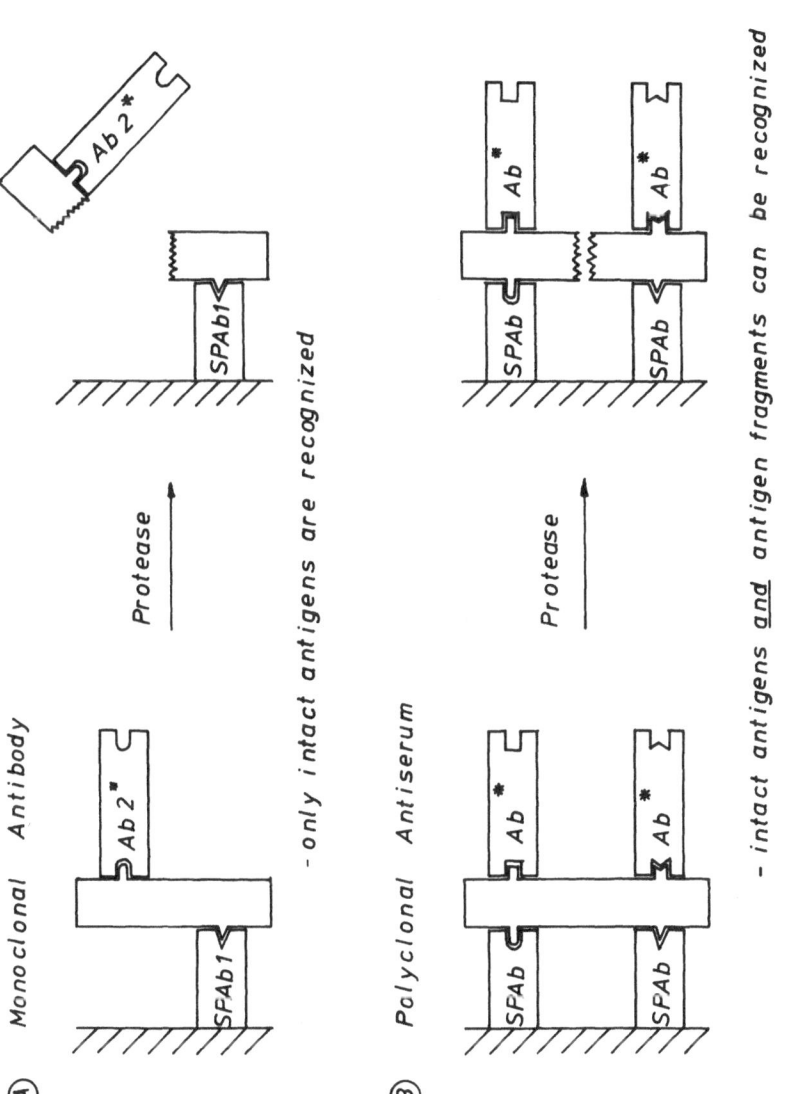

Figure 11.8 Proteolysis

REFERENCES

1. Köhler, G. and Milstein, C. (1975). Continuous cultures of fused cells secreting antibody of predefined specifity. *Nature*, **256**, 495
2. Eisen, H. N. and Siskind, G. W. (1964). Variations in affinities of antibody during the immune response. *Biochemistry*, **3**, 996
3. Siskind, G. W. and Benacerraf, B. (1969). Cell selection of antigen in the immune response. *Adv. Immunol*, **10**, 1
4. Jarvis, M. R., Casperson, G. F., Kranz, D. M. and Voss, E. W. (1982). Affinity maturation of NZB and Balb/cV mice. Antifluorescyl response. *Molec. Immunol.*, **19**, 525
5. Moyle, W. R., Anderson, D. M. and Ehrlich, P. H. (1983). A circular antibody–antigen complex is responsible for increased affinity shown by mixtures of monoclonal antibodies to human chorionic gonadotropin, *J. Immunol.*, **131**, 1900
6. Thompson, R. J. and Jackson, A. P. (1984). Cyclic complexes and high avidity antibodies. *TIBS*, **9**, 1
7. Richards, F. F., Konigsberg, W. H., Rosenstein, R. W. and Varga, J. M. (1975). On the specificity of antibodies. *Science*, **187**, 130
8. Lane, D. and Koprowski, H. (1982). Molecular recognition and the future of monoclonal antibodies. *Nature*, **296**, 200
9. Lennox, E. S. (1983). What can we learn about molecular homologies from cross-reactions of monoclonal antibodies. *Transpl. Proc.*, **15**, 45
10. Sperling, R., Francus, T. and Siskind, G. W. (1983). Degeneracy of antibody specificity. *J. Immunol.*, **31**, 882
11. Berzofsky, J. A. and Schechter, A. N. (1981). The concepts of cross-reactivity and specificity in immunology. *Molec. Immunol.*, **18**, 751
12. Haaijman, J. J., Deen, C., Kröse, C. J. M., Zijlstra, J. J., Coolen, J. and Radi, J. (1984). A jungle of pitfalls. *Immunol. Today*, **5**, 56

12
Monoclonal antibodies: developments in immunocytochemistry

D. ARMELLINI, A. MASSONE, A. TIEZZI,
P. LEONCINI, P. RUGGIERO, M. BUGNOLI,
G. SCAPIGLIATI and V. PALLINI

The origins of immunocytochemistry can be traced back to the development of techniques for the labelling of antibodies with tags visible under the microscope. A close operational link between biochemistry and cytology was thus established, consisting of a classical, three-step experimental design: biochemical purification of individual molecular species (antigens) from tissues; production of antisera; identification of the molecular species *in situ*, exploiting an antigen–antibody reaction. In this procedure the specificity of the cellular staining is clearly based on the specificity of the antisera, which is in turn determined essentially by the purity of the antigen preparation.

The monoclonal antibody (MA) technique[1] has introduced a highly innovative experimental design in immunocytochemical studies, extending, or even shifting, the specificity-determining operation from the preparation of the antigen to the preparation of the antibody. Since all antibodies produced by a single cell line are of a single molecular species, cloning hybridomas is equivalent to isolating immunoglobulins capable of recognizing unique antigenic determinants (epitopes). Epitopes frequently consist of distinct molecular moieties or of limited stretches in a polymer chain. MA thus bring the staining specificity to levels unattainable with polyclonal antisera, and can be prepared by immunization with unpurified antigens, even with whole cells.

Properly selected MA have been, and will continue to be, employed in immunocytochemical research for purposes which can be schematically described as follows:

1. Distinction between structurally related antigens, e.g. homologous polypeptides differing only in limited regions of their amino acid sequence.
2. Recognition of molecules unamenable to purification in immunogenic amounts or of biochemically uncharacterized antigens. This situation is frequently encountered with cellular components which are first defined on a morphological or functional basis.

Following these guidelines we will describe some MA obtained in our laboratory. We will also describe data published in the literature which we believe are representative of the major achievements and of the future trends in diagnostic immunocytochemistry; we will limit our attention to diagnostic problems whose solution has been, or could be, possible only by exploiting the potentialities of the hybridoma-cloning technique. Finally, we will outline some criteria for the selection and characterization of MA intended for use in diagnostic immunocytochemistry.

Different cell types frequently contain specific forms of enzymes (isozymes) which catalyse essentially the same reaction and are structurally related to the point of exhibiting cross-reaction with polyclonal antisera. However, it is well known that immunological distinction among different isozymes can help solve a number of diagnostic problems. Our group has recently been involved in the production and characterization of a panel of MA reacting selectively with the prostatic isozyme of human acid phosphatase. The antibodies have been selected using a solid phase radioimmunoassay; their specificity for the isozyme of normal and neoplastic prostatic epithelium has been further assessed by staining sections of formalin-fixed, paraffin-embedded human organs[2].

The MA technique can be successfully used in all cases of cell- or tissue-specific forms of homologous proteins. We have been able to distinguish human chorionic somatomammotropin (hCS), a placental hormone, from human growth hormone, a pituitary product, both of which exhibit approximately 85% homology in their amino acid sequence. Antibodies specific for hCS have been selected and characterized in their affinity constants in a solid phase assay system[3]. Their use in immunocytochemical studies has been evaluated by staining sections of hormone-producing tissue[4].

The epitope-specificity of MA can be further exploited in the distinction among allelic forms of isozymes and isoproteins[5]. These achievements can be successfully applied in the diagnosis of certain inherited diseases.

The elucidation of the protein composition of the intracellular 10 nm filaments (intermediate filaments, IF) has recently aroused much interest among pathologists. IF are cytoskeletal structures whose electron microscopic appearance is uniform in all cell types, still consist of cell-specific proteins, i.e. of vimentin in mesenchymal cells, of keratins in epithelia, of desmin in muscle cells, of 'neurofilament polypeptides' in neurones, of 'glial fibrillary acidic protein' (GFA) in astrocytes and in Bergmann glia. The cell specificity of intermediate filament protein is usually maintained upon neoplastic transformation and in tumour metastasis[6,7].

It is therefore possible to determine unequivocally the histogenesis also for poorly differentiated tumours by staining sections with antibodies specific for the various IF proteins, provided that their specificity is high enough to avoid cross-reactions. IF proteins form a family of different, but homologous polypetides[8] and cross-reactions do frequently occur with polyclonal antisera. Commercially prepared anti-vimentin antisera have been found to be contaminated with antibodies to keratins[9]; we have repeatedly observed the same and related cases of cross-reaction by testing antisera on fixed cells or electrophoretically separated IF polypeptides. The difficulties in obtaining strictly specific antisera may be due to common epitopes or to impurities present in the antigen preparation, even when it is judged homogeneous by sodium dodecylsulphate (SDS)–polyacrylamide gel electrophoresis. These difficulties can be overcome with monoclonal antibodies recognizing polypeptide-specific epitopes (e.g. Refs. 10, 11). Anti-IF monoclonal antibodies have been reported to be so selective as to detect different phosphorylation states of IF and keratin- or vimentin-associated epitopes which become accessible only during definite phases of the cell cycle or motile activity[12–15]. These and similar MA represent specific probes for cell functional attitudes which may eventually prove to be useful in defining pathological conditions.

The diagnosis of infectious pathogens represents a further field in which the specificity of MA has recently been exploited. Since most micro-organisms have numerous phylogenetic similarities with common antigens, polyclonal antisera tend to react with a wide spectrum of species or types, including pathogenic and non-pathogenic varieties. An immunological distinction of pathogenic *Neisseria gonorrhoeae* and *Chlamydia trachomatis* has recently been obtained with MA which do not react with closely related, non-pathogenic species[16,17]. Human Herpes virus types 1 and 2 can be distinguished by immunofluorescence with monoclonal antibodies with no less sharpness and much more convenience than by analysis with restriction endonucleases and DNA probes[18]. In these cases staining with MA was specific enough to be performed directly on primary clinical specimens, with considerable time-saving over procedures requiring the culture of the micro-organism. The impact of MA in the diagnosis of human infectious diseases has recently been reviewed[19,20].

We have previously reported that MA are epitope-specific probes which can be prepared without previous purification of the antigen. Both properties are conveniently exploited in the immunocyto-chemical study of keratins. Keratins are a numerous family of polypeptides (about 20 components) which form intermediate filaments in epithelial cells. Keratin polypeptides can be satisfactorily purified only in minute amounts by bidimensional polyacrylamide gel electrophoresis; using MA, the existence of both polypeptide-specific and common epitopes was observed (e.g. Refs. 21, 22). Figure 12.1 describes one MA prepared in our laboratory which was obtained by immunization with the whole group of human epidermal keratins; this antibody is directed against one epitope shared by two electrophoretic components of approximately 50 kilodalton, which are expressed only in the basal layer of human epidermis. Such antibodies can be used to study the expression of specific polypeptides in differentiating cells, in primary and metastatic tumours and in various pathological conditions of keratinized epithelia (e.g. Refs. 9, 24–26).

The motile apparatus of cilia (axoneme) from respiratory epithelia consists of about 200 polypeptides (Fig. 12.2). This figure describes two MA obtained by immunization of mice with whole tracheal axonemes, which recognize selectively different axonemal poly-peptides separated by SDS–polyacrylamide gel electrophoresis; immunofluorescent staining of tracheal cells with these antibodies indicates that the described polypeptides are localized in different regions of the ciliary apparatus. We are currently engaged in the selection of MA against discrete axonemal components with the aim of studying the polypeptide phenotype of human cilia from cases of primary ciliary diskinesia, a genetically determined disease character-ized by morphologically and functionally abnormal cilia[27-29].

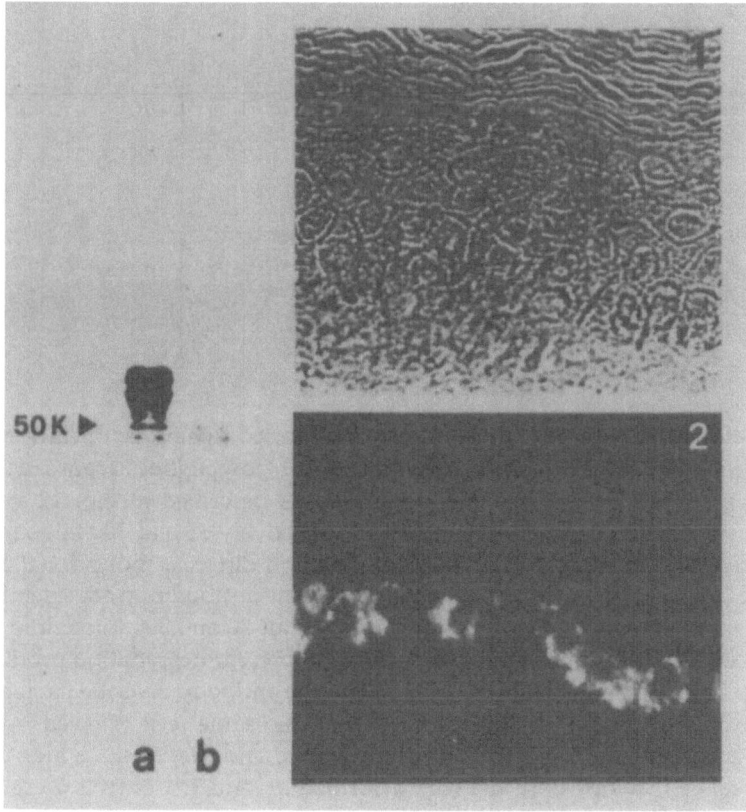

Figure 12.1   Characterization of an MA against human epidermal keratins. (a) Coomassie blue staining of polypeptides from human epidermis; electro-phoresis is performed on 4–16% polyacrylamide gradient gel containing sodium dodecylsulphate in a discontinuous buffer system[47]. (b) Immunoblot with the MA; electrophoretically separated polypeptides have been transferred onto a nitrocellulose sheet and stained by an indirect immu-noperoxidase method[48]. (1) Ethanol-fixed, paraffin-embedded section of normal human skin viewed under Nomarski optics. (Original magnification ×128). (2) Same section as (1); indirect immunofluorescent staining of the epidermal basal layer with the MA. No staining was observed replacing the MA with an immunoblot-negative hybridoma supernatant

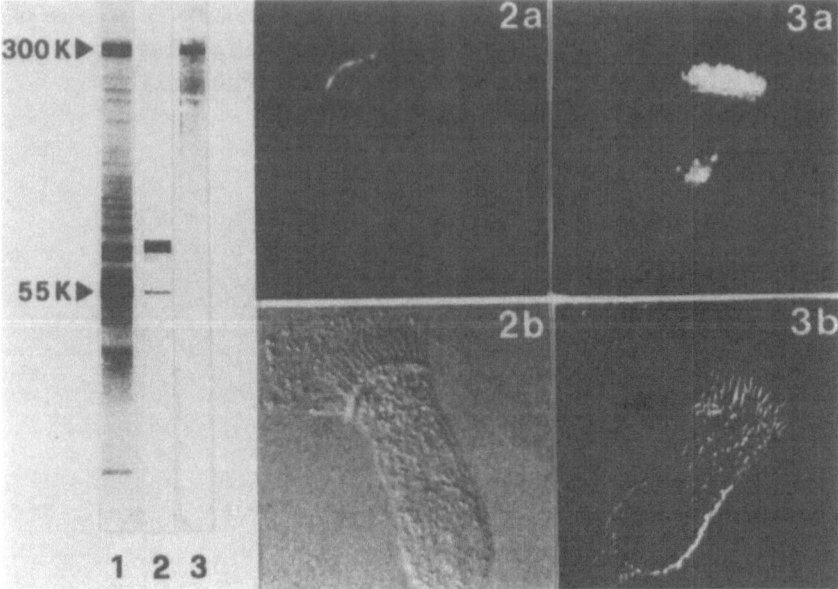

Figure 12.2 Characterization of two MA raised against axonemes from tracheal cilia. (1) Coomassie blue staining of polypeptides from tracheal axonemes. Electrophoresis was performed as described in Fig. 12.1; the migration of tubulin and dynein bands (respectively 55 and 300 kilodalton) is indicated. (2) and (3) Immunoblots with two different monoclonal antibodies, performed as described in Fig. 12.1. The antibodies react essentially with single electrophoretic components of about 70 and 300 kilodalton and stain slightly faster migrating bands which represent degradation products. (2a,b) Staining of detached tracheal cell by the antibody described in lane 2; (2a) indirect immunofluorescence; (2b) the same cell viewed under Nomarski optics. (3a,b) Indirect fluorescence and Nomarski optics on a tracheal cell stained with the MA described in lane 3. Controls were performed as described in Fig. 12.1. (Original magnification ×320)

The importance of MA in determining the progress of modern biology is best exemplified by the characterization of cell type or cell function-associated antigens whose very occurrence was defined only by indirect approach. In these instances immunization is usually performed with whole cells or cell fractions and MA selected by morphological or physiological assay systems can eventually be instrumental in the purification and molecular characterization of the antigen. This procedure clearly reverses the sequence of operations imposed upon immunocytochemical studies by the use of polyclonal antisera. As to one significant result achieved through this novel experimental design, we make reference to the first biochemical characterization of the T lymphocyte antigen receptor by means of MA specific for individual T cell lines (e.g. Ref. 30). Operationally similar research trends based on MA include the study of antigens involved in cell adhesion and metastasis (e.g. Refs. 31, 32) or expressed typically in proliferating cells[33,34], which will conceivably produce basic scientific knowledge, also of use in the diagnosis and prognosis of neoplastic and displasic lesions. In this connection it is interesting to report that the determination of the cell proliferation index via a monoclonal antibody against bromodeoxyuridine, an artificial DNA precursor, has become a significant procedure in tumour analysis[35,36]. Up to now, however, the greatest impact upon diagnostic immunocytochemistry has been exerted by MA specific for tumour-associated antigens and for markers of white blood cell development and differentiation. The various diagnostic uses of these antibodies have recently been reviewed[37-39]. MA will conceivably continue to be the main tool for the identification of tumour-associated antigens; the recent development of an efficient procedure for the immunization of human patients with autologous tumour cells permits interesting developments in this area of research[40].

MA also tend to replace polyclonal antisera in routine immunocytochemical analyses because they can be more conveniently used and produced. In fact, staining of tissues and cells with MA usually results in a higher signal-to-noise ratio, and hybridoma lines are a virtually inexhaustible source of antibodies with defined characteristics, whereas the properties of antisera may be difficult to reproduce.

There are, however, unfavourable consequences of the hybridoma-cloning procedure, which demand a proper characterization of MA intended for immunocytochemical use. One unpleasant consequence is the specificity of a single MA for an epitope which is in itself 'unspecific', i.e. it is shared by different antigen molecules[41]. In these cases the MA will not be a specific probe, as can be checked by staining electrophoretic bands on nitrocellulose blots or cellular structures in immunomicroscopic observations. Such antibodies may be more frequently met in cases in which the unspecific epitope is located in an 'immuno-dominant' region of the molecule chosen for immunization. It is conceivable that these difficulties can be overcome by immunizing with selected molecular moieties, e.g. oligopeptides, obtained by cleavage or chemical synthesis.

On the other hand, a single epitope is sometimes not enough to diagnose certain cell types, e.g. all strains of pathogenic gonococci or all cases of a certain tumour[19,42]. In these cases, false-negative results can be avoided by using relatively small groups ('panels') of MA with different specificities.

The chemical structure of antigens may be modified or destroyed by the various fixation procedures necessary in immunocytochemical analyses (e.g. Refs. 43–46). Different epitopes may be differently affected by these procedures. As a consequence it is advisable that characterization of MA includes a description of their specificity in terms of polypeptides and cellular structures, and also precise recommendations about fixation methods and other conditions of use.

REFERENCES

1. Köhler, G. and Milstein, C. (1975). *Nature*, **256**, 495–7
2. Cianfriglia, M. *et al.* (1984). *J. Exp. Clin. Cancer Res.*, **3**, 49–52
3. Mariani, M. *et al.* (1984). *J. Immunol. Methods*, **71**, 43–8
4. Neri, P. *et al.* (1983). In Peeters, H. (ed.) *Protides of the Biological Fluids*. Vol. 31, pp. 1067–70
5. Harris, H. (1983). *Ann. Rev. Genet.*, **17**, 279–314
6. Osborn, M. and Weber, K. (1983). *Lab. Invest.*, **48**, 372–94
7. Denk, H. *et al.* (1983). *Am. J. Pathol.*, **110**, 193–208
8. Geisler, N. and Weber, K. (1982). *EMBO J.*, **1**, 1649–56
9. Erlandson, R. A. (1984). *Am. J. Surg. Pathol.*, **8**, 615–24
10. Gown, A. M. and Vogel, A. M. (1984). *Am. J. Pathol.*, **114**, 309–21
11. Osborn, M., Debus, E. and Weber, K. (1984). *Eur. J. Cell Biol.*, **34**, 137–43
12. Sternberger, L. A. and Sternberger, N. H. (1983). *Proc. Natl. Acad. Sci.*, **80**, 6126–30
13. Franke, W. W. *et al.* (1983). *J. Cell Biol.*, **97**, 1255–60
14. Franke, W. W. *et al.* (1984). *Exp. Cell Res.*, **154**, 567–80
15. Dulbecco, R. R. *et al.* (1982). *Proc. Natl. Acad. Sci.*, **80**, 1915–18
16. Stephens, R. S. *et al.* (1982). *J. Immunol.*, **128**, 1083–9
17. Tam, M. R. *et al.* (1982). *Infect. Immun.*, **36**, 1042–53
18. Goldstein, L. C. *et al.* (1983). *J. Infect. Dis.*, **147**, 829–37
19. Nowinski, R. C. *et al.* (1983). *Science*, **219**, 637–44
20. Engleberger, N. C. and Eisenstein, B. I. (1984). *N. Engl. J. Med.*, **311**, 892–901
21. Woodcock-Mitchell, J. R. *et al.* (1982). *J. Cell Biol.*, **95**, 580–8

22. Tseng, S. C. G. *et al.* (1982). *Cell*, **30**, 361–72
23. Gigi, O. *et al.* (1982). *EMBO J.*, **1**, 1429–37
24. Cianfriglia, M. *et al.* (1984). *J. Exp. Clin. Cancer Res.*, **3**, 49–52
25. Leoncini, P. *et al.* (1984). Abstract no. 176, International Symposium on Monoclonal Antibodies: Biological and Clinical Applications. Florence
26. Weiss, R. A., Eichner, R. and Sun, T.-T. (1984). *J. Cell Biol.*, **98**, 1397–1406
27. Tiezzi, A. *et al.* (1984). Abstract no. 123, International Symposium on Monoclonal Antibodies: Biological and Clinical Applications, Florence
28. Afzelius, B. A. (1979). *Int. Rev. Exp. Pathol.*, **19**, 1–43
29. Sleigh, M. A. (1983). *Eur. J. Resp. Dis.*, **64**, (Suppl. 127), 157–61
30. Samelson, L., Germain, R. and Schwartz, R. (1983). *Proc. Natl. Acad. Sci.*, **80**, 6972–6
31. Oesch, B. and Birchmeier, W. (1982). *Cell*, **31**, 671–9
32. Vollmers, H. P. and Birchmeier, W. (1983). *Proc. Natl. Acad. Sci.*, **80**, 3729–33
33. Rao, P. N. (1984). Abstract SG-10-6, 3rd International Congress on Cell Biology, Tokyo
34. Sato, C. *et al.* (1984). *Exp. Cell Res.*, **155**, 33–42
35. Dulbecco, F. *et al.* (1983). *Proc. Natl. Acad. Sci.*, **80**, 5573–7
36. Morstyn, G. *et al.* (1983). *J. Clin. Invest.*, **72**, 1844–50
37. Sell, S. and Wahren, B. (eds.) (1982). *Human Cancer Markers.* (Clifton, N.J.: Humana Press)
38. Fink, L. M. and Clarke, S. M. (1984). *Prog. Clin. Pathol.*, **9**, 121–33
39. Bernard, A., Boumsell, L., Dausset, J., Milstein, C. and Schlossman, S. F. (eds.) (1984). *Leucocyte Typing.* (Berlin: Springer Verlag)
40. Hoover, H. C. *et al.* (1984). *Cancer Res.*, **44**, 1671–6
41. Lane, D. and Koprowski, H. (1982). *Nature*, **296**, 200–2
42. Kemshead, J. T. *et al.* (1983). *Lancet*, **1**, 12–15
43. Altmannsberger, M. *et al.* (1981). *Lab. Invest.*, **45**, 427–34
44. Pinkus, G. S. (1982). *Human Pathol.*, **13**, 411–15
45. Kaku, T. *et al.* (1983). *Am. J. Clin. Pathol.*, **80**, 806–15
46. Stein, H. *et al.* (1984). *Lancet*, **2**, 71–3
47. Laemmli, U. K. (1970). *Nature*, **227**, 680–5
48. Towbin, H., Staehlin, T. and Gordon, T. (1979). *Proc. Natl. Acad. Sci.*, **76**, 4350–4

Part 4
BIOSENSORS

13
Technical aspects of biosensors

A. K. COVINGTON

INTRODUCTION

Complicated surgical procedures, which are now considered routine, would not be possible without the benefit of present-day patient-monitoring techniques. All monitoring systems rely on a transducer to convert the biological phenomena into electrical data which are then processed and displayed in an appropriate form for the clinician. At present the weakest link in any system is invariably the transducer, the biomedical sensor, or biosensor.

There are many widely differing types of biosensor in use, ranging from the simple chloridized silver strips used to detect electrical activity of muscles and the brain (EMG, ECG, EEG), to the more complex types such as infra-red absorption cells for the determination of expiratory P_{CO_2}, and newer developments of electrochemical devices such as ion-selective and enzyme electrodes. Clinical usage imposes extraordinarily stringent demands with regard to precision, stability and safety, but ergonomic and economic factors are also important. Three distinct modes of operation common to all biosensors can be identified:

1. *In-vivo*: the sensor is implanted or introduced percutaneously; there are great difficulties with sterilization procedures which may compromise the biosensor function.
2. On-line (*ex-vivo*): the sensor is connected directly to the patient, but in a non-invasive manner; the sampling rate can be made small and non-return.
3. *In-vitro*: the sensor is used discretely without any connection to the patient; i.e., in an analytical laboratory instrument, with resulting problems of sample storage and delay in results becoming available.

NEW TECHNIQUES

Recent important developments for clinical science include:

1. Ion-selective electrode instrumentation for the analysis of body fluids, whole blood, plasma, serum, and urine for sodium, potassium and calcium[1]. In this area, flame photometric methods have been dominant but sophisticated microprocessor-based ion-selective electrode instrumentation for these ions is taking its place beside pH and blood-gas analysers. The advantages over flame methods are speed, sample size and possibility of development of *in-vivo* instrumentation. Since the normal range of blood cations is so small, high precision is necessary; for example for sodium only a 2.4 mV change is involved at 37 °C. For other ions of clinical interest, Mg^{2+}, HCO_3^- and Cl^-, no adequate sensor materials are available yet.

2. Enzyme electrodes[2]. This term in general use is a misnomer since they are complete electrochemical cells. They can be used to detect glucose, urea, lactate, pyruvate and other blood metabolites making use of amperometric or potentiometric detection of the product of an enzymic reaction. The enzyme is immobilized in a membrane over the surface of the electrochemical sensor and a second permselective membrane is often used to protect the enzyme from deleterious contact with whole blood. These devices, being dependent on diffusion of substrate in and product out of the membrane, tend to be slow in response.

3. Microelectronic chemical sensors or chemical-sensitive field effect transistors (ChemFETs) have been successfully used[3,4] for the direct analysis of blood electrolyte cations (hydrogen, sodium, potassium, calcium) with the use of on-line indwelling cannula sampling[5]. This *ex-vivo* cannula approach has the advantage of precise, continual monitoring with the small size of devices permitting connections to the patient with minimal dead space, providing fresh, reliable physiological data without the difficulties associated with *in-vivo* measurement. These devices are integrated circuit (IC) chips comprising four enhancement mode, dual dielectric ChemFETs and four insulated gate FETs. The devices are encapsulated to form part of a miniature flow-through cell which is incorporated into a remote sensor head containing a miniature

valve assembly, allowing blood or a calibration solution to be passed through under microcomputer control[3]. The ion-sensitivity is provided by silicon nitride for hydrogen ions, valinomycin for potassium and by synthetic neutral carriers for sodium and calcium[6]. The system has been successfully tested for potassium ion analysis[4] and more recently four-function devices have been developed and tested and used for on-line *ex-vivo* blood analysis[7]. Problems of calibration are of paramount importance.

CALIBRATION

All electrochemical sensors require calibration and, depending on their stability, often fairly frequent recalibration. The reasons and the principles involved will be illustrated with reference to the ion-sensors, ion-selective electrodes (ISEs), now widely used in clinical analysers for sodium, potassium, and calcium ion determinations in whole blood, serum, plasma and urine. Measurement of unknown ion concentration is made by determining the change in potential difference of an ISE reference electrode pair when transferred between a calibration standard solution and an unknown. This change in potential difference (ΔE) between the two solutions is given by the Nernst equation as:

$$(\Delta E = (k/z_i)\,\Delta\log a_i$$

where k is the theoretical slope factor, $RT(\ln 10)/F$ (61.5 mV at 37 °C), and a_i is the activity of the ion i of charge z_i. This equation assumes that there are no changes at any other site of potential difference in the cell below during the measurement.

Ag | AgCl | KCl + AgCl ‖ Calibration | ISE | Internal | AgCl | Ag
or   filling
unknown   solution
solution

As in pH measurements, there is assumed to be no change in liquid junction potential when one solution is replaced by another. This idealized situation is never achieved in practice, and changes can be expected when solutions differ in ionic strength, composition, pH and, for clinical samples, in protein and erythrocyte content.

The magnitude of such errors is basically unknown, although attempts at estimation are made. Their effect can be minimized by choosing the calibration solution to be similar in most respects to the unknown. The method of forming the liquid junction is also important since the junction geometry affects the potential across the junction. Memory effects can be observed from diffusion of previous solutions into the porous membranes usually used in construction of restricted flow reference electrodes. Two solutions differing by 4% in concentration of a monovalent ion would show a potential difference change of only 1 mV between an ISE responsive to that ion, and a reference electrode transferred between the two solutions. For a divalent ion the change would be only 0.5 mV. It is therefore necessary for clinical purposes to measure to 0.1 mV.

The advent of the microprocessor has greatly increased the sophistication of many of the instruments now becoming available and, as with other microprocessor instrumentation, the meaning of the output signal, and more important here, its significance to the clinician, is not always clear. ISEs respond to ionic activity in solution, that is to free ions and not to bound or complexed ions. However, if an instrument is calibrated with an ionic concentration calibration standard, closely matching the unknown, it will yield the concentration of the sensed ion in the unknown solution. Although some activity standards have been proposed, they have not been generally adopted. Some companies seek to give the clinician values to which he is accustomed, so the values given by an ISE instrument for sodium and potassium are often adjusted by choice of composition of the calibration standard solution, or by software correction, to be in accordance with flame photometer values. Some companies offer a choice of scales. A further complication is whether the results should be expressed in terms of actual volume of the sample or in terms of plasma water, a 7% difference. Difference between these various scales is called bias. For ionic calcium determination the situation is more complex since only about half of the total calcium is ionized and half protein-bound or complexed; only the former is sensed by the ISE.

OUTLOOK

The whole situation is confused, and evidence suggests that the variation of results between samples run on different instruments is much greater than desirable. Such variations can arise from the ISE, from liquid junction effects, or from incorrect software corrections or other sources. Standardization is urgently needed, and is actively under consideration by the European Working Group for Ion-Selective Electrodes (EWGISE) of IFCC under the chairmanship of A. H. J. Maas (Utrecht).

REFERENCES

1. Covington, A. K. (1982). Ion-selective electrodes in clinical medicine. *Med. Lab. World*, **7**, 11–17
2. Vadgama, P. (1984). Enzyme electrodes for continuous in-vivo monitoring. *Trends Anal. Chem.*, **3**, 13–16
3. Covington, A. K. and Sibbald, A. (1985). Microelectronic chemical sensors for chemical analysis. Proceedings of NBS Meeting on Direct Potentiometric Measurements on Blood, Washington DC, USA, May 1983 (In press)
4. Sibbald, A., Covington, A. K., Cooper, E. A. and Carter, R. F. (1983). On-line measurement of potassium in blood by chemical-sensitive field effect transistors: a preliminary report. *Clin. Chem.*, **29**, 405–6
5. Janata, J. and Huber, R. J. (1980). Chemically sensitive field effect transistors. In Freiser, H. (ed.) *Ion-selective Electrodes in Analytical Chemistry*. pp. 107–74. Vol. II. (New York: Plenum Press)
6. Simon, W., Ammann, D., Anker, U. Q. and Band, D. M. (1984). In Shinton, N. K. (ed.) *New Technologies in Clinical Laboratory Science*. pp. 115–22. (Lancaster: MTP Press)
7. Sibbald, A., Covington, A. K. and Carter, R. F. (1984). Simultaneous on-line measurement of blood potassium, calcium, sodium and pH by use of four-function ChemFET integrated circuit sensor. *Clin. Chem.*, **30**, 135–7

14
Ion selective electrodes and their clinical application in continuous ion-monitoring

W. SIMON, D. AMMANN, P. ANKER,
U. OESCH and D. M. BAND

INTRODUCTION

Ion selective electrodes (ISE) are devices that permit the activity of a given ion in a solution to be determined potentiometrically despite the presence of other ions. The general layout of an ISE cell assembly has been previously reviewed[1,2]. A great number of ISE have been developed and recommended for analytical application[2]. Undoubtedly, the fundamentally different types of membranes offer a host of attractive applications in the field of selective ion detection[1,2], yet the potential of liquid membrane electrodes is virtually unlimited[1]. They allow the construction of cell assemblies in a wide variety of shapes and sizes[1,3]. Examples are dip-in macroelectrodes[3], microelectrodes (tip diameter $\leqslant 1\,\mu m$)[4], catheter electrodes[5-10], surface electrodes[11,12], ion selective field effect transistors (ISFET)[13-15], flow-through assemblies[3,15] and potentiometric analysis slides[16]. The neutral carriers especially, defined as ionophores that carry no charge if not complexed by the selected ion, have led to ISE with a large range of selectivities[1,3]. Here we report on the use of neutral carrier-based solvent polymeric membranes[17] for the continuous monitoring of ion activities in whole blood.

OPTIMIZED ION SELECTIVE ELECTRODES

The clinical application of ISE imposes severe demands in respect to selectivity, stability of the measured cell potential difference (EMF),

Table 14.1 Requirements for potentiometric ion-activity determinations and related performance of optimized membrane electrodes

Ion I^{z+}	Concentration range (mmol/l)	Activity range (mmol/l)	EMF range (mV)	Tolerable standard deviation[a] (mV)	Measured EMF stability[b] (mV)
Na^+	135–150	102–112	2.4	0.12	0.06
K^+	3.5–5.0	2.6–3.7	9.1	0.46	0.11
$Ca^{2+,c}$	1.0–1.2	0.34–0.41	2.4	0.12	0.11
H_3O^+	4.3×10^{-5}–5.6×10^{-5}	3.34×10^{-5}–4.35×10^{-5} (pH 7.48–7.36)	6.8	0.35	0.37

[a] For a 5-fold subdivision of the given physiological range with a 95% confidence limit
[b] EMF change of an aqueous calibration solution before and after 6h of continuous measurement in blood of the extracorporeal circulation
[c] Free ionized Ca^{2+}

response time and life-time of the electrodes[1,3]. Table 14.1 indicates a very narrow expected EMF range (column 4) for the specified physiological range (columns 2 and 3) of Na^+, K^+, Ca^{2+} and H_3O^+. A reasonable resolution within this range demands standard deviations in the EMF measurement smaller than those indicated in column 5 of Table 14.1. In view of this goal, the plasticized poly(vinyl chloride) membranes presented in Table 14.2 (for membrane components see Figure 14.1) have been studied in the extracorporeal blood bypass of dogs and rabbits[18].

Table 14.2 Optimized membrane compositions for continuous measurement in whole blood

Membrane for Ion I^{z+}	Composition (wt.%) (see Figure 14.1)
Na^+	1.2% ETH 227; 66.3% ETH 469; 32.5% PVC
K^+	1.3% valinomycin; 68.3% ETH 469; 30.4% PVC
Ca^{2+}	3.3% ETH 1001; 2.1% KTpClPB; 63.7% ETH 469; 30. 9% PVC
H_3O^+	1.0% Tridodecyl amine; 0.5% KTpClPB; 65.6% ETH 469; 32.9% PVC

RESULTS AND DISCUSSION

The membranes presented in Table 14.2 have been used in a previously described flow-through system[19]. The system was calibrated before and after contact with blood. Runs lasting 6 h or more for the simultaneous continuous measurement of Na^+, K^+, Ca^{2+} and H_3O^+ in the extracorporeal blood bypass of dogs and rabbits yielded EMF shifts of the calibration solution before and after the run of only 0.06 mV (Na^+), 0.11 mV (K^+), 0.11 mV (Ca^{2+}), and 0.37 mV (H_3O^+)[18]. A comparison of columns 5 and 6 in Table 14.1 indicates that the membranes presented in Table 14.2 indeed have the required stability. Therefore there is no need for an intermediate calibration over periods of at least 6 h. The selectivity of the membranes is sufficient to avoid corrections for interfering ions present in whole blood[1,3,18]. In permanent contact with whole blood a continuous use

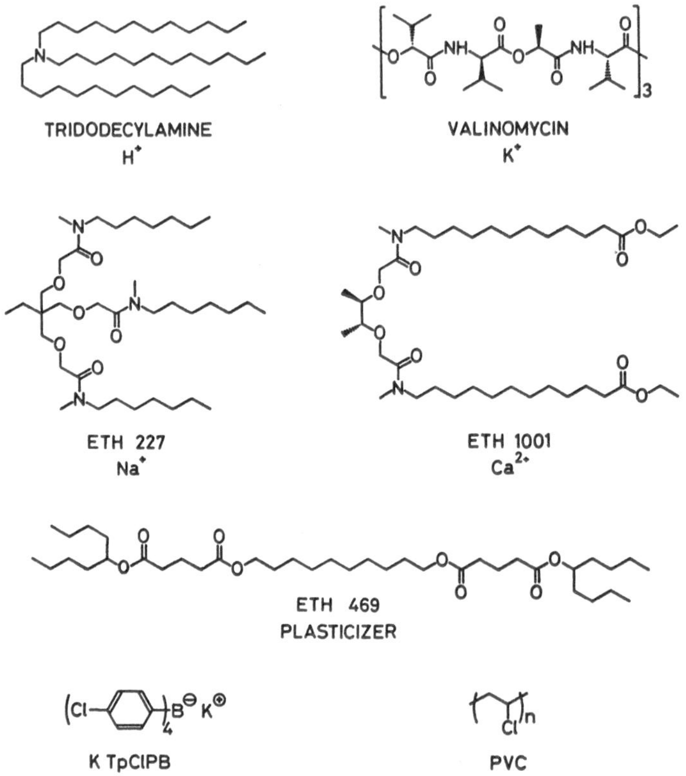

Figure 14.1   Constitutions of the membrane components discussed

life-time of membranes of the type specified in Table 14.2 longer than 3 months[1,3,20] can be expected.

Neutral carrier-based membranes containing valinomycin[23] and tridodecyl amine[24] respectively have been used in catheter electrodes. The simultaneous recording of the K^+-concentration and pH is shown for such electrodes in Figure 14.2. The catheter electrodes, of a diameter of about 1 mm, were passed into the abdominal aorta of an anaesthetized cat via a femoral artery. KCl was then injected via the femoral vein. The effect on the arterial potassium is seen as a sudden rise to about 9 mmol/l followed by a fall and a smaller recirculation peak. The effect of the sudden gross change in potassium is to stimulate the carotid body chemoreceptors, the nervous discharge from which produces a very large breath. This in turn results in a sudden fall in the carbon dioxide level of the arterial blood, and a consequent fall in hydrogen ion activity is recorded by the pH sensing catheter.

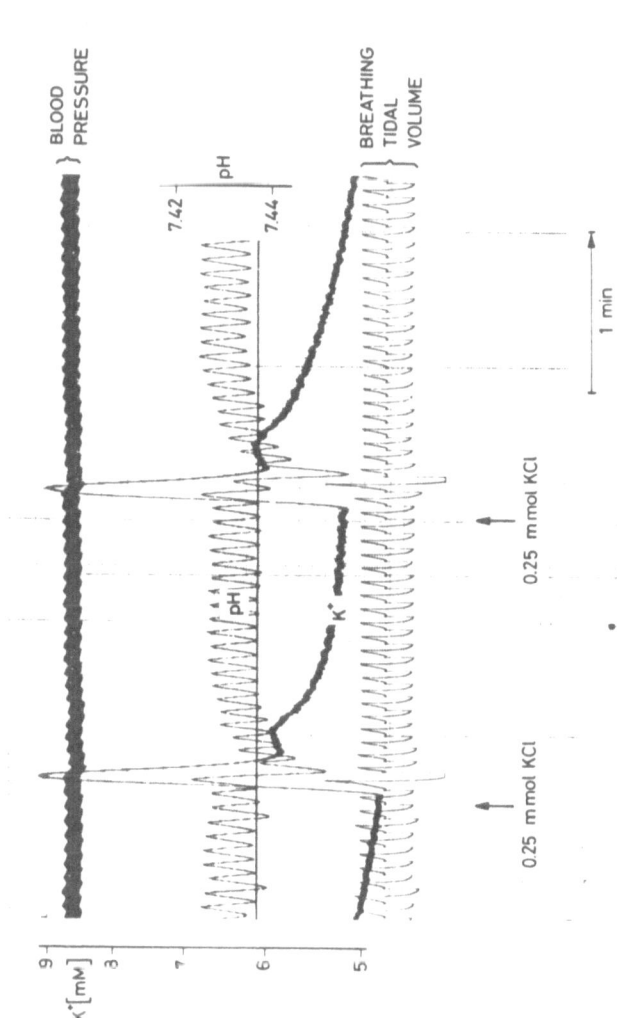

Figure 14.2 Arterial blood K$^+$ concentration and pH recorded continuously in the abdominal aorta of an anaesthetized cat using solvent polymeric membrane catheter electrodes

The pH catheter electrode operated for several hours without deterioration of the electromotive behaviour. This is a major advance over the glass electrodes, the performance of which deteriorates rapidly, probably as a result of protein deposition on the membrane. The pH records were made using a voltage-to-frequency converter which was optically isolated from the main recording equipment. The potassium trace was obtained with a radio-telemeter probe unit[25]. The catheters had separate reference electrodes connected to the blood via saline bridges.

OUTLOOK

The highly selective and reliable potentiometric systems now available for the determination of Na^+ and K^+ metal cations are likely to displace flame photometry in clinical laboratories in the next few years[3]. Neutral carrier-based sensors for a wide variety of other cations (e.g. Li^+)[3], including organic ions, are at hand. Enantiomer-selective systems are entering analytical relevance[21]. Neutral carriers for anions open up a large variety of accessible selectivities for anion selective sensors[22].

ACKNOWLEDGEMENTS

This work was partly supported by the Schweizerischer National-fonds zur Förderung der Wissenschaftlichen Forschung. One of us (P.A.) thanks Rhône-Poulenc for a grant.

REFERENCES

1. Meier, P. C., Ammann, D., Morf, W. E. and Simon, W. (1980). Liquid-membrane ion-selective electrodes and their biomedical applications. In Koryta, J. (ed.) *Medical and Biological Applications of Electrochemical Devices.* pp. 13–91. (Chichester, New York, Brisbane, Toronto: John Wiley & Sons)
2. Freiser, H. (ed.) (1978). *Ion-selective Electrodes in Analytical Chemistry.* Vols. 1 and 2. (New York, London: Plenum Press)

3. Ammann, D., Morf, W. E., Anker, P., Meier, P. C., Pretsch, E. and Simon, W. (1983). *Ion-Selective Electrode Reviews*, **5**, 3–92
4. Thomas, R. C. (ed.) (1978). *Ion-Sensitive Intracellular Microelectrodes*. (London, New York, San Francisco: Academic Press)
5. Band, D. M., Kratochvil, J., Poole Wilson, P. A. and Treasure, T. (1978). *Analyst*, **103**, 246–51
6. Lim, M., Linton, R. A. F., Wolff, C. B. and Band, D. M. (1981). *Lancet*, **2**, 591
7. Lim, M., Band, D. M. and Linton, R. A. F. (1981). *Crit. Care Med.*, **9**, 181
8. Treasure, T. (1978). *Intens. Care Med.*, **4**, 83–9
9. Schindler, J. G. and Gülich, M. v. (1981). *Biomed. Technik*, **26**, 43–53
10. Hill, J. L., Gettes, L. S., Lynch, M. R. and Hebert, N. C. (1978). *Am. J. Phys.*, **235**, H455–9
11. Wiegand, V., Güggi, M., Meesmann, W., Kessler, M. and Greitschus, F. (1979). *Cardiovasc. Res.*, **13**, 297–302
12. Hirche, H., Franz, C. and Bös, L. (1979). Ion-selective electrodes in cardiac ischemia. In Zülch, K. J. *et al.* (eds.) *Brain and Heart Infarct*. Vol. II, pp. 104–11. (Berlin, Heidelberg, New York: Springer Verlag)
13. Moss, S. D., Janata, J. and Johnson, C. C. (1975). *Anal. Chem.*, **47**, 2238–43
14. Janata, J. and Huber, R. J. (1980). Chemically sensitive field effect transistors. In Freiser, H. (ed.) *Ion-Selective Electrodes in Analytical Chemistry*. pp. 107–74. (New York, London: Plenum Press)
15. Sibbald, A., Covington, A. K. and Cooper, E. A. (1983). *Clin. Chem.*, **29**, 405–6
16. Hamblen, D. P., Glover, C. P. and Kim, S. H. (1977). US Patent 4,053,381; Battaglia, C. J., Chang, J. C. and Daniel, D. S. (1980). US Patent 4,214,968
17. Moody, G. J., Oke, R. B. and Thomas, J. D. R. (1970). *Analyst*, **95**, 910–18
18. Ammann, D., Anker, P., Metzger, E., Oesch, U. and Simon, W. (1985). Continuous potentiometric measurement of different ion concentrations in whole blood of the extracorporeal circulation. In Kessler, M. *et al.* (eds.) *Ion Measurements in Physiology and Medicine*. pp. 102–10. (Berlin, Heidelberg, New York, Tokyo: Springer Verlag)
19. Anker, P., Wieland, E., Ammann, D., Dohner, R. E., Asper, R. and Simon, W. (1981). *Anal. Chem.*, **53**, 1970–4
20. Oesch, U., Dinten, O., Ammann, D. and Simon, W. (1985). Lifetime of neutral-carrier based membrane in aqueous systems and blood serum. In Kessler, M. *et al.* (eds.) *Ion Measurements in Physiology and Medicine*. pp. 42–7. (Berlin, Heidelberg, New York, Tokyo: Springer Verlag)

21. Bussmann, W. and Simon, W. (1981). *Helv. Chim. Acta*, **64**, 2101-8
22. Wuthier, U., Pham, H. V., Zünd, R., Welti, D., Funck, R. J. J., Bezegh, A., Ammann, D., Pretsch, E. and Simon, W. (1984). *Anal. Chem.*, **56**, 535-8
23. Band, D. M., Kratochvil, J. and Treasure, T. (1977). *J. Physiol.*, **265**, 5P-6P
24. Schulthess, P., Shijo, Y., Pham, H. V., Pretsch, E., Ammann, D. and Simon, W. (1981). *Anal. Chim. Acta*, **131**, 111-16
25. Band, D. M., Cowell, T. K. and Treasure, T. (1979). *J. Physiol.*, **293**, 14P

Index

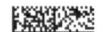